MIND Diet

for

Beginners

The Complete Guide to Improving Your Brain Health and
Preventing Dementia, Alzheimer's, and Other Diseases

IVAN BURROWS

IVAN BURROWS

MIND Diet for Beginners

ISBN: 9798372653481

IVAN BURROWS

Table of Contents

IVAN BURROWS

Introduction

W e are at a point in our lives where science and technology have been able to cure several illnesses that have plagued humanity for several years. However, there are still many sicknesses and diseases that science and technology have not been able to determine the exact cause or solution to, and the rate of new illnesses is skyrocketing. Therefore, we can strive for good health by considering our diet. Our health is in our hands, and it is time for every one of us to take charge of our lives by using our food and nutrition to beat diseases and transform our health. Some scientific evidence has shown that certain foods cause specific illnesses, while others help prevent them. Is that not great? Knowing full well that all you need to do is stay away from unhealthy foods and stick to the beneficial ones. Even though consuming a healthy diet does not guarantee 100% good health, it, however, decreases your likelihood of contracting some of these diseases, unlike others who consume these harmful foods.

The biggest threat to humanity is not communicable diseases but non-communicable diseases like stroke, heart disease, cancer, diabetes, obesity, and neurodegenerative conditions. And I am pretty sure you know someone who has had one of these illnesses. According to the World Health Organization, non-communicable diseases kill about 41 million people every year; cardiovascular disease accounts for most non-communicable diseases, with about 17.9 million people dying every year, followed by 9.3 million people dying of cancer annually, 4.1 million people dying from chronic respiratory diseases, and 2.0 million people dying of diabetes. Even with all the treatments and breakthroughs for all these illnesses, they are not a sustainable solution for non-communicable diseases. Drug treatment alone cannot keep us healthy. We have to do our own part in maintaining our health. That is why I have decided to put down all I know in this book.

I am a certified nutrition, strength, and conditioning specialist, a certified personal trainer, and a sleep science and health certificate holder. I am also a nutrition and wellness consultant certificate holder, a mind-body medicine certification program graduate, and a Mediterranean diet certificate holder. I decided to pursue these courses as I realized the importance of demonstrating my expertise beyond my research and knowledge. The idea of this book starts as a reflection of my life's soul-searching journey and how I was able to find medicines within my kitchen. This course just added credibility and expertise in the field. We are what we eat, and what we feed our bodies determines how physically and mentally fit we become. I sincerely hope that this book helps you, the reader, to delve deeper into the wonders of food and how our gut plays a major role in our health. Often, the medicines we think we need are already in our kitchen cabinet and can address daily problems like obesity, acidity, bloating, depression, heart disease, thyroid disease, brain disease, and even cancer. Sometimes all you have to do is take a deep breath, drink enough water, and get out in the fresh air instead of loading your stomach with drugs from the hospital.

This book has been written in a way that will make it easier for you to understand the vital role food plays in your physical and mental health. MIND Diet for Beginners: The Complete Guide to Improving Your Brain Health and Preventing Dementia, Alzheimer's, and Other Diseases is not just any other type of book, but it is unique because I have penned down my experience and years of research so that you will have a nourishing and healthy life. I saw dementia and Alzheimer's disease cases in my family, and that's why I believe in the power of our diet and how our gut influences us. This book is packed with the tools and information you need to make better decisions about your food. After reading this book, you will be more convinced that the ice cream in your freezer or the candy on your table poses a significant threat to your health. This book caters to everyone; if you are healthy and fit and want to continue in good health, this book is for you; if you are starting to feel your age and you want to prevent a decline in your health, this book is for you; if you have any autoimmune disease or a chronic condition, this book is for you.

The information I have packed in this book isn't intended to replace medical care. I am not against Western medicine, and I believe that medical technology is just as important as the food we consume. This book is to guide you, whether you are healthy or sick. There is no "one shoe size" that heals all illnesses and leads to longevity. That is, no single thing in our lives would prevent sicknesses. But there is a way to improve and boost the immune system so the body can repair and heal itself. Having a good immune system gives you a better chance of fighting and defending your body from various sicknesses. The decisions you make on food throughout your life will determine your health. The best decision to make is to start your health journey as soon as possible and not wait till you are older and your body is not functioning like it used to. Your diet is an extra step to maintaining a healthy and balanced life. A good diet, regular exercise, stress management, and quality sleep can help you attain your full health potential.

A healthy diet produces a healthy brain. Cognitive decline is increasingly common these days and, if left unchecked, may eventually lead to death. The MIND diet is a diet for your brain health, and if you have not heard about the MIND diet, this book contains so much information about the diet, even for beginners. It is common knowledge that what you put on your plate can either improve or hinder your cognitive abilities, such as your memory, attention, language, etc. This book will show you how easy it is to maintain a sharp and healthy brain with just a proper and healthy diet.

If I had been privileged to know what I know now when I was much younger, I would have avoided so many things. I am grateful that I have this knowledge now, and that's why I am more than willing to share this knowledge with anyone and everyone willing to know more about their health. I don't want you to make the same mistakes I made when I was younger. So, I have taken the time to give you a step-by-step guide to healthy living through a healthy diet. With this book, you will understand more about food and your health and how great food impacts your physical, mental, and emotional well-being. You cannot continue to spend so much money on drugs when you can easily eat to beat the several diseases out there.

IVAN BURROWS

BOOK 1

IVAN BURROWS

Chapter One

———— ··•·· ————

How Food Impacts Your Health

What does food have to do with our health? Food plays an essential role in our lives, and we must treat what we eat with care. Basic science tells us that food gives the body the energy needed to build and rebuild cells, which is necessary to prevent sicknesses and keep the human body healthy. As humans, we need all the nourishment we can get to sustain a healthy life, and some of this nourishment comes from food. Food is considered one of the necessities of every living being, alongside water, shelter, clothing, air, safety, and sleep. Unlike other plants and animals, humans have a wide variety of food options, which are frequently defined by geography, culture, religion, and personal preference. Your eating habits, to a large extent, determine your health.

Understanding What Health Truly Means

How should your health be taken care of? Is food directly proportional to how the body functions? What constitutes good health? Generally, good health is the absence of sicknesses and diseases. Many people do not fully understand what health means. Some people believe that if you feel or look good, you are healthy. Others believe that you are in perfect health if you show no symptoms. However, this is not entirely true. The World Health Organization describes "health" as a complete state of physical, social, and mental well-being and not just the absence of infirmity and diseases.

Furthermore, the World Health Organization sees health as a tool for everyday life. This means a person can be physically fit but mentally unfit due to stress, anxiety, and worries. Your overall health includes physical, mental, emotional, social, and environmental health. Therefore, having good health should not be underestimated.

Food and Nutrients

Food is any substance that is taken and consumed and interacts with the body to create and repair tissues, supply energy, and control biological processes. Food comes in several forms: liquid, solid, simple, and complex. Simple food means eating a single meal, while complex food means eating several foods.

Food consists of two components: nutrients and non-nutrients. The nutrients in our food play a vital role in our health, and having the right combination of nutrients is essential for healthy living. Food nutrients are grouped into carbohydrates, protein, fats, vitamins, minerals, and water. If these nutrients are not present in our food, our health will decline. Nutrients provide instructions for our body to function healthily. They are the nourishing substances present in food that are essential for our growth and development. It's essential to understand what foods to include or exclude from your diet. Scientists have discovered that our food is linked to specific health problems such as heart disease, diabetes, cancer, depression, etc. To live a healthy life, one needs to understand how these multiple nutrients interact to help the body function properly.

On the other hand, the body does not always require non-nutrients present in the diet to function properly. They are nutrients that can be made by the body or absorbed from food eaten. They are also known as non-essential nutrients. Examples of non-nutrients obtained from food include probiotics, prebiotics, dietary fiber, antioxidants, and certain amino acids. Therefore, healthy food consists of both nutrients and non-nutrients in the appropriate composition.

What makes food healthy? While it might be challenging to define what food belongs to a healthy food, one should know that whatever food you choose should be adequate. Food adequacy means that the food eaten should provide all the nutrients the body needs to function correctly. The amount and frequency of the foods need to be considered to determine if the food is adequate. Secondly, the food eaten has to be balanced in terms of nutrient composition. There is also a recommended daily allowance or intake of food nutrients that humans need. Thirdly, the food calories should be controlled. This means that humans need a certain level of calories to maintain a healthy lifestyle. Measuring the calorie intake of people can be done using several formulas. The number of calories you should eat per day depends on numerous factors, including your age, sex, height, current weight, activity level, and metabolic health, among several others. But if we follow recommendations from the US Department of Agriculture's Dietary Guidelines for Americans, then:

Woman:

- between the ages of 19–30 require 2,000–2,400 calories per day to maintain their weight
- between the ages of 31–59 should consume 1,800–2,200 calories per day to maintain their body weight
- over the age of 60 require fewer calories, around 1,600–2,000 calories per day, to maintain their weight

Men:

- between the ages of 19–30 should consume 2,400–3,000 calories per day to maintain their weight
- between the ages of 31–59 need about 2,200–3,000 calories per day to maintain their weight
- over 60 generally requires 2,000–2,600 calories

Keep in mind that the exact number of calories may vary depending on factors such as your activity level, height, weight, health status, and other factors.

It's also important to create a calorie deficit if you're trying to lose weight. This can be done by consuming fewer calories than you normally do or by exercising more. Some people even choose a combination of both, eating fewer calories and being more physically active for better and quicker results.

Diet

Diet refers to the variety of foods that you consume. A good and healthy diet should constitute healthy foods (such as vegetables, water, and whole grains) that promote good health and restrict or limit those seen as risky or unhealthy (such as salt, sugar, and fat). These foods can come from different sources, such as vegetables or animals.

Healthy Food Consistency

Eating a single food with poor nutrient content once or twice will not significantly affect your health unless it becomes a habit. The same goes for healthy food as well. Healthy eating will not start to have a positive impact on your life until it becomes a routine. One or two portions of ice cream, for instance, won't have a substantial effect on your health. However, consuming ice cream consistently for more than a year can have detrimental effects on your health.

Consistency is vital when it comes to eating the right food to foster good health. Food consistency means eating healthy every time or most of the time. What is considered "most of the time" may differ from person to person. You have to decide what is appropriate for you.

Here are some tips for adopting healthy food consistency:

- Understand what healthy food is: The first step is to determine what a healthy meal is. There are many misconceptions about what constitutes a healthy meal, so be aware of what you're eating. Processed foods do not count as healthy foods.

- Know and respect your body: Understand how your body works and learn what foods it likes and dislikes. Eating foods that your body dislikes might cause disruption and confusion in its internal system.

- Plan your meals: Knowing what you're going to eat in advance can save time and make it easier to maintain healthy eating habits. This can be bought or cooked food, and investing in containers and a fridge to store food can be helpful.

- Strike a balance: Eating a balanced diet means including a variety of food groups in a day, which can help you maintain food consistency.

- Eat natural foods, go organic, and eat more greens: Eat foods like fruits, salads, and vegetables. You can grow vegetables in your garden. Choose foods that are free from unnatural or naturally occurring toxins. Unnatural toxins can come from poor food handling or genetically modified food, whose effects on humans are not yet understood.

- Display healthy foods in conspicuous places: Sometimes, it is best to place healthy foods like fruits and nuts in prominent places instead of storing them in the fridge, so they are easily accessible. You can do this by putting some fruits in a bowl next to the door or on the dining table so that you can quickly grab them before you go out.

- Spice up your diet with various foods: The brain craves novelty, so it is best to vary your diet to keep things interesting.

Why do You Crave Junk Foods?

Junk foods, such as packaged chips, donuts, and french fries, have been linked to a variety of health problems, including heart-related diseases, obesity, high blood pressure, and other health problems. However, many people still consume unhealthy food despite the knowledge and information out there about how unhealthy food negatively affects the body.

- Our brains and sugar: Humans have been programmed to go for the sweeter food than the bitter food.

- Junk food is designed to trigger cravings: Many things are considered when preparing junk foods. The smell, taste, and mouthfeel are one of the most critical factors used to perfectly engineer junk food. For example, the crunchiness of the chips and the fizziness of sodas have been analyzed numerous times to cause consumers to become addicted. These foods are prepared to get you hooked so that you will keep coming back to eat more and more.

- Stress affects your relationship with food: When you are exposed to a long period of stress, a hormone called cortisol is released, which damages the way you think about food. This hormone causes people to be drawn to fattening "comfort foods", which have a soothing effect on stress by curbing brain activity in the stress centers. However, this is only temporary. Even when this effect wades off, it becomes too late to stop the triggering because the brain has made the connection with these foods as foods that calm our nerves.

We all need food as living beings, but the relationship between food and our health is not as straightforward as some people may believe. It is important to understand the appropriate types and quantities of food to consume. Consuming too much food, too little food, or the wrong type of food will harm your health. That is why you must understand the relationship that exists between food and your health. Poor nutrition is one of the significant contributors to morbidity and is linked to more than one in four deaths in the US. Many people develop chronic diseases related to poor-quality food or dietary patterns. This means that food plays a significant role in helping people live healthier lives and also contributes to premature death.

It is also important to understand the relationship that people have with food. Not everyone might be able to make the switch from consuming unhealthy food to healthy food. This can be because not all healthy and quality foods are equally accessible. Also, more nutritious food items like fruits and vegetables are generally more expensive than junk foods. Furthermore, modifying people's consumption habits is quite difficult because people's eating habits are hard to change. Eating habits are complex and influenced by factors such as evolution, cultural identity, social relationships, family, and psychology. As a result, most people do not have complete control over what they eat.

Several factors, such as price, nutrition, convenience, taste, pleasure, satiety, healthfulness, medicine, familiarity, weight, dietetics, tradition, marketing, hedonism, ethical concerns, etc., can influence eating habits. Researchers have found that taste is one of the significant driving factors influencing what people eat, as people are not likely to compromise the taste of their food for a health benefit.

Importance of Food (How it Nourishes the Body)

Nutrition knowledge is essential to make health-conscious decisions when it comes to food. If you do not know something, then you are bound to make mistakes. Knowledge about nutrition plays a crucial role in promoting healthier food habits which leads to a healthier body. People who are aware of the consequences of poor nutrition are likely to follow a healthy diet. However, this is not always the case because some people continue to eat unhealthy foods even when they are aware of the negative effects on their health. However, nutritional knowledge can be an excellent way to promote healthy living.

The first thing to know about food is to understand the food classes. Food contains carbohydrates, proteins, fats, vitamins, minerals, and water. Food taken into the body is digested and converted into nutrients that are utilized by the body.

Fats

Saturated Fatty Acids

Butter, tallow, coconut, and suet (cows and lambs), lard from pigs, and fats from geese, chicken, turkey, and ducks are saturated fats. They are all referred to as traditional dietary fats since they have all been used for cooking for ages before commercially saturated fats like margarine and shortening were developed. Naturally, saturated fats are usually solid at room temperature. They include different fatty acids like lauric acid (coconut and palm kernel oil), palmitic acid (butter, cocoa butter, olive oil, soybean oil, meat, and sunflower oil), butyric acid (animal fat, plant oils, butter, and parmesan cheese), myristic acid (dairy products), and stearic acid (cocoa butter and meat). These fatty acids have antifungal, antibacterial, and anti-inflammatory properties that protect the body.

There are many misconceptions about saturated fatty acids, and some believe that saturated fats are dangerous. However, there are many benefits to eating saturated fats. Saturated animal fats obtained from pasture-fed livestock produce vitamins A, D, and K2. Saturated fats lower heart disease risks, they help stimulate prostaglandin three, a pain-reducing anti-inflammatory that exerts a protective effect that is mediated through the anti-inflammatory and cholinergic pathways by activating the nicotinic acid receptors and cholecystokinin. The body can produce saturated fats through refined carbohydrates if you are not eating enough fats.

Trans Fatty Acids

Trans fatty acids are also known as trans-fat or trans-unsaturated fatty acids. They naturally occur in small amounts in milk, fat, and meat. They grew in popularity in the early 20th century from an unintended by-product in the industrial processing of vegetable and fish oils for use in margarine and later in packaged baked goods, snack foods, and fast food. The high temperature used in the hydrogenation of liquid vegetable oils breaks down vegetable fats to create trans fat. Using hydrogenated oils to cook would result in the food being high in trans fats. It is advisable to avoid using unhealthy oils or trans fatty acids and use healthy oils to cook to enhance brain function. Scientific evidence reveals that even minimal amounts of trans fat consumed can interfere with the delta-6 desaturase enzyme and other enzymes needed to transform omega-3 and omega-6 into essential fatty acids required for life sustainability and cellular and organ health. Essential fatty acids are required by the body but cannot be synthesized by the body and must be obtained from dietary sources.

Polyunsaturated Fatty Acids (PUFAs)

The human body cannot produce PUFAs, but they are needed for the body to function properly; one must get PUFAs from their diet. They include corn oil, sunflower oil, soybean oil, and fatty fish such as tuna, salmon, mackerel, herring, and sardines. Oils containing PUFAs are usually liquid at normal room temperature and solid when cooled. Also, leafy greens, nuts, fish, and seeds contain polyunsaturated fats.

Omega-3 and omega-6 are the two types of essential fatty acids that are obtained from polyunsaturated fats. Omega-9 can also be derived from polyunsaturated fats as a non-essential fatty acid because the body can convert omega-3 and omega-6 to omega-9.

Even though polyunsaturated fats are low in saturated fats and are cholesterol-free, they easily become toxic and rancid when used for frying and can easily cause inflammation. Also, polyunsaturated oils are known to cause liver damage, sterility, lung damage, weight gain, digestive disorders, impaired immune function and reproductive health, and neurological problems.

Monounsaturated Fatty Acids (MUFAs)

MUFAs are a type of unsaturated fat. They are healthy oils derived from vegetable sources such as tree nuts, avocados, and olives. There are several types of MUFAs, such as oleic, palmitoleic, and vaccenic acids. Oleic acid is the most common type of MUFA, and 90% of oleic acid can be found in the diet. Many foods contain high amounts of MUFAs, but they are mostly a combination of different fats. It is just a few foods that contain only one type of fat.

Foods high in unsaturated fats, such as olive oil, are generally liquid at room temperature. In contrast, foods with a high concentration of saturated fats, like coconut oil and butter, are typically solid at room temperature. Olive oil is popularly known for its medicinal value on the gall bladder and its abundant chlorophyll source, which helps detoxify the intestinal tract. Other healthy foods containing MUFAs include:

- Red meat from beef and lamb.
- Wildlife like elk, bear, and moose.
- Full-fat dairy products.

Essential Fatty Acids (EFAs)

EFAs are essential to health and are obtained from foods. The primary essential fatty acids include omega-3 (linolenic acid), omega-6 (linoleic acid), and Arachidonic acid (AA). Fish oils such as cod, salmon, sardine, and krill should be incorporated into your diet for brain and memory.

Carbohydrates

Foods rich in carbohydrates generate energy for the body and regulate fat metabolism. Carbohydrates comprise sugar molecules that are either simple or complex. A simple sugar (carbohydrate or starch) consists of a single molecule, while a complex sugar (carbohydrate or starch) consists of many sugar molecules bonded in a chain. Sugar is the simplest form of carbohydrate and can be found in refined sugar, dairy products, fruits, and vegetables. Complex carbohydrates are either fiber or starch. Starch sources include carrots, potatoes, wheat, barley, rice, oats, chips, cornstarch, and certain dessert foods. Carbohydrates are broken down into glucose before the body can utilize them.

Proteins

Proteins are good for physical and mental health. They can be derived from animal and plant sources and fuel every function of living cells. Some animal proteins include fish, beef, whey, eggs, and casein, while plant proteins include hemp, peas, soy, and rice. Before the body can utilize protein, it must break it down into amino acids through digestion.

Everyone has different protein requirements relative to their biochemistry. Some people require more protein than others and vice versa. However, stressful times will require more protein as proteins help to repair the body. Generally, men need more protein than women. Also, humans require more protein during physical exercise.

Protein deficiency is not usually caused by inadequate protein intake but the inadequate digestion of protein. Poor protein digestion is caused by insufficient hydrochloric acid, which helps to break protein down. Insufficient hydrochloric acid causes a reduction in nutrient absorption, protein not fully digested, and impaired satiety signal to the brain. The use of antacids also causes protein deficiency.

People on a strict vegetarian diet who do not eat plant protein are most likely to have protein deficiency. Symptoms of protein deficiency include slow wound healing, fatigue, hair loss, lack of mental focus, impaired immune function, and emotional instability.

Chapter Two

•———— ··•·· ————•

How Stress Affects

Digestion

Digestion is the process in which food is broken down into smaller particles to be absorbed into the bloodstream and utilized by the body. Stress affects gastrointestinal function, and for one to have smooth digestion, stress has to be eliminated. Stress causes problems like indigestion, constipation, diarrhea, heartburn, nausea and vomiting, and lower abdominal pain. Stress can be physical or mental, and they activate the brain's stress response systems which in turn harm the body. It is important to note that stress has adverse effects on the body's major systems are affected by stress (sweat glands, muscular, cardiovascular, and urinary). Stress is one factor that has not been given enough attention when maintaining good health and preventing diseases. Most attention has been on regular physical activity and adequate nutrition, neglecting how stress can bring about severe health problems.

Digestion

The gastrointestinal (GI) tract is a long system of hollow organs combined to create an intact tube that begins at the mouth and stops at the anus. These organs include the mouth, esophagus, stomach, small and large intestines, rectum, and anus. Also, there are additional solid organs that help in the digestion process, and they include; the liver, gall bladder, and pancreas.

When food enters the mouth, it is chewed and broken down by saliva. The saliva adds a lubricating antibacterial fluid that assists the food in traveling down the esophagus. The food leaves the esophagus and travels into the stomach. The stomach contains powerful acids that break down food so it can be easily absorbed. The liver and gall bladder help in the digestion of fats. The pancreas contains pancreatic juices rich in enzymes that wash foods, and then the washed foods are referred to as chyme. Foods not fully broken down can become fermented in the digestive tract. For example, if vegetables are placed inside a covered pot, and a fire is not ignited to cook the vegetables, they start to ferment and become sour over time. Also, there will be bubbles, and it will start to smell. This happens in the stomach of someone who cannot digest their food properly. This will lead to bad breath and flatulence.

The digestive enzymes in the body can be likened to a fire on a stove that helps to cook food that can be eaten. These enzymes help in the breaking down of foods into nutrients that the body can absorb. The salivary glands, stomach, pancreas, and intestine all secrete digestive enzymes. These enzymes can also be found in raw foods like papaya, pineapple, etc. Food intolerances may result from deficient enzyme levels. The digestion process begins in the mouth. Here, starch is broken down by chewing and mixing the food with the salivary enzymes. The process ends in the colon with the excretion of waste. Also, cooked foods are more easily digested than raw foods.

It is important to chew your food properly. The advice says to chew your food an estimated 32 times before swallowing. This appears to be an average number applied to most bites of food. Foods that are harder to chew (such as steak, nuts, etc.) may require up to 40 chews per mouthful. Soft and water-filled food like watermelon may require as few as 10 to 15 chews. The goal of chewing is to break down your food, so it loses texture.

Stress can affect digestion, starting from the way you chew your food. If you chew your food hurriedly, large chunks of food will be passed to the esophagus, which will be unprepared for further digestion. Stress can also occur at the esophageal sphincter. Due to stress, it might get opened when it is not supposed to be opened and closed when it should not be closed. Sometimes, it might relax too much and close on the part of the stomach which pushes the stomach up. This condition is called a hiatal hernia. Stomach acid rises into the lower esophagus if the esophageal sphincter does not close effectively. And this will lead to gastroesophageal reflux disease (GERD) or acid reflux. Studies have found high rates of GERD in people suffering from PTSD, which shows there is a relationship between GERD and anxiety.

People chew food rapidly when they are stressed, and this makes them swallow larger chunks of food. When stressed, the acids and enzymes needed to break down food cannot perform their job. Indigestion in the stomach leads to the development of pain and gases, which causes nutrients to be malabsorbed and organs in the body to be malnourished. Therefore, it is advisable to eat food slowly because it makes it easier for starch to be broken down. The enzyme amylase stored in the salivary glands is used to store carbohydrates as they are secreted to aid in the digestion of sugars. There are two kinds of saliva; the thin, watery saliva used to moisten the food and mouth, and the thick mucus saliva used to lubricate the form and form it into a ball called bolus which can be swallowed.

The stomach receives the food which the salivary enzymes could have predigested. Stomach acid helps in the digestion of proteins because proteins are large food molecules that are required to be broken down by proteolytic enzymes into smaller molecules called amino acids, which are, in return, building blocks of the neurotransmitters. The stomach muscles help to churn the food up to combine it with gastric juices. Therefore, food cannot be digested in the absence of stomach acid. This is another way that stress can affect the digestion process. Pepsin secreted in the stomach begins the protein digestion process. The pancreas also secretes trypsin, chymotrypsin, proteases, and proteolytic enzymes into the small intestine. The proteolytic enzymes secreted into the small intestine assist in the breaking down of the protein that the stomach has not fully digested. The absence of pancreatic enzymes will lead to the non-absorption of proteins and fats, and this can lead to nutritional deficiencies.

Stomach secretions are made up of stomach acid (hydrochloric acid), many enzymes, and a mucus coating to protect the stomach lining. Low-level or insufficient hydrochloric acid or gastric acid secretion is known as hypochlorhydria. Hypochlorhydria causes undigested food to enter the small intestine and colon, which makes it unusable for the body. The gut will no longer be able to use the NTs like tryptophan and tyrosine required for healthy neurotransmitter production for the brain. This can lead to asthma, pain, depression, anxiety, food allergies, and severe indigestion.

The production of this acid reduces with age and can lead to digestive problems such as small intestinal bacteria overgrowth (SIBO) due to raised pH levels. SIBO impedes the absorption and assimilation of nutrients like vitamins B6, B12, and B vitamins folate, which causes anxiety and depression. Therefore, poor digestion leads to poor mental health.

If hypochlorhydria is left untreated, it can lead to several chronic health issues.

Symptoms of Low Stomach Acid

- Stomach upset
- Gas, bloating, burping, belching, flatulence
- Undigested food in stool

- Desire to eat when not hungry
- Brittle fingernails
- Hair loss
- GI infections
- Iron deficiency
- Fatigue
- Severe candida infection
- Vision changes
- Numbness
- Adult acne
- Some Causes of Low Stomach Acid
- Stress- chronic stress is known to cause a reduction in the production of hydrochloric acid in the stomach.
- Age- hypochlorhydria occurs mostly in older people, especially adults above 65 years.
- Vitamin Deficiency- a deficiency in B vitamins and zinc can cause low stomach acid. The deficiencies may be caused by inadequate dietary intake or nutrient loss from alcohol consumption, smoking, and stress.
- Medications- some medications taken over a long time can cause hypochlorhydria. Antacids or medications used in the treatment of ulcers and acid reflux, like PPIs.
- Helicobacter Pylori (H. Pylori)- H. pylori is a bacteria that infects the stomach. It can damage the tissues in your stomach

and the first part of your small intestine. H. pylori is very common among people, and a greater population of people will likely have it. Although not everyone who has it shows symptoms, many will show symptoms. These bacteria secrete an enzyme called urease which neutralizes the stomach and causes it to be less acidic. This process weakens your stomach lining and causes your stomach cells to be easily hurt by acid and pepsin, which are strong digestive fluids. H. pylori is one of the major causes of gastric ulcers, and if left untreated, it can cause a decrease in stomach acid. The bacteria can also stick to the stomach cells leading to inflammation.

- Surgery- sometimes, surgeries done in the stomach can lead to gastric bypass surgery, which can lead to the reduction of stomach acid.

The utilization of a supplemental HCL can increase HCL production. Supplemental HCL helps to destroy harmful stomach bacteria, which increases nutrient absorption. Also, copper, iron, zinc, boron, magnesium, calcium, selenium, and vitamins B3 and B12 perform their job effectively.

The gallbladder helps to emulsify fats required to elevate mood, reduce stress, reduce inflammation, and maintain artery health. The brain is mostly made of docosahexaenoic acid, and neurons need fats to function effectively, just like cars require lubrication to function properly. If the body cannot use or have access to good fat, it can lead to the brain not getting enough fuel. If the gallbladder malfunctions, fish oil supplements or dietary fats will not be effective enough because the nutrients cannot be emulsified and assimilated.

Naturally, the liver and the gallbladder work as a team to emulsify fat. The bile in the gallbladder consists of salts, lecithin, and cholesterol esters. It helps to emulsify and separate fats into smaller fat globules to be able to pass through the digestive system. A low-fat diet can slow down the gall bladder's muscle motor. The muscle motor helps to push bile into the duodenum, and when it fails, it can lead to a build-up of sludge. Alcohol abuse, refined foods, junk food, and Trans fatty acids lead to chronic gallbladder congestion, gallstones, gravel, and low bile output. Other symptoms of gallbladder problems include flatulence, burping, shoulder pain, nausea, etc.

Most cholesterol can be found in the liver, and adequate cholesterol is vital for mental health. Although there is a worldwide view that cholesterol is not good, sufficient cholesterol is essential for the functionality of the brain and nervous system. When insufficient amounts of cholesterol are not obtained from food, the body tries to maintain a balance by producing more cholesterol. Also, the total amount of body cholesterol decreases when you consume quantities of cholesterol more than what the body needs. Many believe cholesterol is a significant cause of heart disease, but this is not always true. Using medications and diets that are extremely low in fats to reduce cholesterol will lead to mental distress, anxiety, muscle pain, and suicide attempts.

Cholesterol is a precursor of hormones, the raw material used to produce some fat-soluble vitamins like vitamin D. It is used to repair arterial inflammation, mainly caused by stress, contamination from waste, Trans fats, environmental toxins, and manufactured food. Reducing inflammation is one of the best ways of managing one's cholesterol and not reducing or eliminating cholesterol. Restricting the cholesterol in your diet will simultaneously decrease the quantity of Omega-3 in the diet and DHL. Omega-6 levels in the body continue to increase, and this causes an imbalance in the ratio between omega-3 and omega-6 levels. Therefore, this alters the brain tissues and raises an individual's vulnerability to depression.

Cholesterol is vital for vitamin D synthesis, which is a fat-soluble vitamin. Studies have found that a deficiency in vitamin D leads to depression and chronic pain. Also, cholesterol is a precursor for glucocorticoids which are crucial for blood-sugar regulation, blood pressure regulation, ligament strength, mineralocorticoids for mineral balance, and sex hormones. Also, cholesterol forms the basis for pregnenolone which is a predecessor to almost all other steroid hormones (such as cortisol, progesterone, aldosterone, and testosterone). Low levels of pregnenolone cause anxiety, depression, and pain.

The pancreas is an organ that acts as an exocrine and endocrine gland. The pancreatic juice consists of protein-digesting enzymes called proteolytic enzymes, which break down proteins, starches, and fats. As an exocrine gland, the pancreas secretes digestive enzymes into the small intestine, which helps break down chime, which just left the stomach and entered the duodenum. These pancreatic enzymes contain proteases, trypsinogen, chymotrypsinogen, amylase, and lipase. Lipase is an enzyme that helps in the breakdown of fats, and the salivary gland also secretes it. These vital enzymes help to convert fats into compounds that the body can utilize as fatty acids and glycerol. The pancreas, as an endocrine gland, helps in the production and secretion of hormones into the bloodstream, which helps regulate glucose metabolism and blood glucose levels. These hormones include glucagon, which increases blood sugar, and insulin, which lowers it. Pancreatic enzymes, as well as supplemental proteolytic enzymes, improve mental health by reducing inflammation.

Digested food flows into the small intestine from the stomach. The small intestine works by peristalsis. Peristalsis is a muscle's involuntary, undulating, and wave-like movement that pushes food through the intestine by contraction and relaxation. Stress disturbs the natural peristaltic rhythm, which can lead to complete disruption.

According to Hans Selye, stress is the body's non-specific response to any demand for change. Studies have found that stress affects the digestive system. Stress can lead to the shedding of good microflora. This leads to a lowered defense system which reduces resistance to pathogenic organisms. Stress can also lead to the suppression of mucosal immunity, gastric ulcers, ion secretion, altered gastrointestinal motility, and increased permeability, leading to the movement of antigens to the lamina propria and bacteria translocation.

Chapter Three

Food Diet and The Brain

Mental development is affected by several factors, including nutrition. Numerous research papers indicate the interconnection between optimal brain performance and healthy nutrition. It has been established that food nutrients provide the structural elements that are required to perform a crucial role in DNA composition, cell multiplication, and neurotransmitter and hormone metabolism, which are essential parts of the brain's enzyme systems. Our nutrition plays a vital role in preventing and treating mental disorders. Poor nutrition culminates in and aggravates mental illness. The sudden discovery of nutrition as one of the many treatments for mental disorders has led to the formation of the conceptualization of brain foods. Brain foods are foods that enhance the performance of the brain. Your brain health is not autonomous of your overall health. Whatever is done to cater to your overall health will affect your brain and vice versa. A healthy diet has positive benefits throughout your life cycle, especially as you age because it helps to preserve your cognitive health, which enables you to remember, learn, think, and make decisions.

Epidemiology is the study of how frequently diseases occur in different groups of people and why they happen. It is a subset of medical science that researches the factors that determine the presence and absence of diseases and disorders. Over the years, epidemiological research has examined the relationship between food and brain health and observed that adhering to the Mediterranean dietary patterns, which consists of high consumption of vegetables, fruits, nuts, and legumes; modest consumption of poultry, eggs and dairy products; and infrequent consumption of red meat—helps to reduce depression, cognitive decline, Alzheimer's disease, dementia, and other related mental problems. More information about the Mediterranean diet can be found in the "INTERMITTENT FASTING FOR WOMEN AND MEDITERRANEAN DIET FOR BEGINNERS: The Complete Guide on How to Lose Weight and Increase Longevity" written by

Emma Collins. I found her books very clear and complex written. The DASH (Dietary Approaches to Stop Hypertension) diet is another dietary pattern that is nourishing for brain health, and it is recommended to reduce blood pressure and heart disease risk. The diet includes vegetables, fruits, whole grains, low-fat dairy products, nuts, poultry, and fish.

The Brain

The human brain is designed to interpret sensory input and decipher incoming information, develop short and long-term memories, originate and coordinate most muscular movements, and regulate many of our organ functions.

There are three major parts of the brain: the cerebrum, cerebellum, and brain stem. The largest part of the human brain is the cerebrum, which is responsible for learning, emotions, fine motor control, and correctly interpreting touch, vision, hearing, and memory. The cerebellum and the brain stem control digestion, breathing, body temperature, and balance. The brain consists of the left and right hemispheres, with each of the hemispheres containing four sections. That is one in front, one in the back, and two in the middle, which are stacked over each other.

These sections are called lobes, and they are eight in number. These lobes are associated with a set of instructions, they are dependent on each other, and they do not act alone. Research has shown that multiple brain parts stay active simultaneously during a task.

The front lobe is also called the frontal lobe, and it is the most developed part of the brain. It gathers information from our senses (sight, smell, taste, touch, and hearing) and spatial awareness (balance and movement). The frontal lobe is in charge of planning and understanding abstract ideas, voluntary movement, short-term memory, and expressive language.

The lower middle lobe is also called the temporal lobe. It helps in hearing, learning, memory, understanding language, and retaining information. The upper, middle, and lower regions are referred to as superior, medial, and inferior. The medial temporary lobe (MTL) consists of the hippocampus, which is involved in forming spatial navigation and long-term memories. Damage to the MTL leads to disorientation and memory loss.

The upper middle lobe is also called the parietal lobe. This lobe plays a significant role in making sense of what the body touches. It also plays a crucial role in spatial thinking, like storing ideas of movement, rotating objects in the mind, and controlling intentions to move. It's also involved in short-term memory, like the frontal lobe.

The last and fourth sections are located at the back of the brain. The back lobe is also called the occipital lobe. This part of the brain is farthest from the eyes, yet it plays a significant role in your vision.

The cerebellum is below the back lobe and has more neurons than any other part of the brain. It helps in learning and coordinating movement.

The brain uses up the most energy (up to 20% of your daily calories) than other organs in the body; it is termed the body's hungriest organ. It has a high metabolism, and it uses up nutrients quickly. The brain prefers glucose which is obtained from the breakdown of food.

The brain needs energy and antioxidants. It is sensitive to oxidative stress due to unstable molecules that damage cells or more free radicals than antioxidants to neutralize them. Oxidative stress causes so much damage to the brain tissue. Antioxidants (such as vitamins E, C, and A, enzymes, plant compounds, and flavonoids) and minerals (such as manganese, zinc, selenium, and copper) are needed to save the brain from oxidation and inflammation.

The body uses two kinds of antioxidants; enzymes created by the body and nutrients derived from food. The antioxidant enzymes produced by the body prevent toxic substances from being created in the first place. The antioxidant nutrients derived from foods also help neutralize oxidation's negative effects. Antioxidant nutrients from food have a bigger role to play in the brain because the brain does not have many antioxidant enzymes at its disposal like other parts of the body. Therefore, it is important to eat healthy foods and develop healthy brain development.

The Early Brain

Genotype and environmental factors such as nutrition, social interactions, parental care, stress, and diseases form the foundation for the development as well as the functional makeup of the brain. Early childhood forms the foundation of a child's later years. Nutrition plays an important role in laying the basis for the development and foundation for cognitive development and social-emotional skills during the early stage of brain development. During this period, it is important to adequately feed the child in other to promote optimal brain function. At this stage of a child, any nutritional deficiency will be fatal and will affect the child for the rest of their life if proper measures are not immediately taken.

Healthy nutrition containing adequate proteins, micronutrients, etc., provided at the appropriate time, will ensure the child's smooth and proper brain development. The first three years of a child's life are crucial in developing a healthy brain.

How Micronutrients Influence the First Three Years of a Child

Micronutrients are nutrients that are needed in trace quantities for the development of an organism.

Essential Fatty Acids

Essential fatty acids are referred to as those polyunsaturated fatty acids that the body cannot produce; these nutrients must come from your diet. The human brain is rich in lipids, and essential fatty acids are the key molecules that determine the integrity and ability of the brain to perform; the brain cells cannot function properly without them. There are two classes of Polyunsaturated Fatty Acids (PUFAs). They are the omega-6 and omega-3 fatty acids. The parent omega-6 fatty acid, linoleic acid (LA), is desaturated in the body to produce arachidonic acid. The parent omega-3 acid alpha-linolenic acid (ALA) is desaturated by the microsomal enzyme system through a chain of metabolic steps to produce eicosapentaenoic acid (EPA) and docosahexaenoic acid (DHA).

A diet rich in fatty acids positively affects a child's memory, language, learning skills, and cognitive competence. DHA affects the hippocampus, frontal lobes, and basal ganglia of the brain, which are the fundamental areas of cognitive function. The accumulation of omega-3 fatty acids helps enhance heightened attention, information processing, problem-solving, and improved cognition in children. Inadequate intake of omega-3 fatty acids reduces the DHA in the brain, leading to abnormal brain disorders and brain damage. It can also lead to neurodevelopmental disorders like dyslexia, autism spectrum disorder, and Attention Deficit Disorder-Hyperactivity Disorder (ADHD).

Zinc

Zinc is an essential nutrient needed for the brain, and zinc deficiency appears to be a crucial problem worldwide. Zinc helps regulate diverse metabolic activities in the body, such as DNA and protein synthesis.

Also, it helps with the maturation and migration of neurons, neurogenesis, and synapse formation. Zinc can be found in high concentrations in the synaptic vesicles of the hippocampal neurons, which are primarily known to be involved in learning and memory. Zinc deficiency may increase the blood-brain barrier permeability that protects the brain from several foreign matters and toxic agents. Zinc has antioxidant properties that help to protect this barrier. Also, zinc deficiency can lead to poor attention, learning, and memory capacity.

Iron

Iron is an important nutrient required for all the stages of human development. It is critical for the development of children as it is vital for the fetal brain's normal anatomical development. The most common micronutrient deficiency in children is iron deficiency, which can permanently damage the brain's cognitive function and structure, irrespective of therapies with iron supplements. Researchers have found that iron deficiency leads to delayed motor development by ten months of age, delayed cognitive processing by ten years, and poorer emotional health as one approaches mid-twenties.

Iodine

Iodine is an important trace element used for the biosynthesis of thyroid hormones and the functioning, development, and increase of metabolism throughout a person's life. An iodine deficiency can cause mental retardation and permanent brain damage. Globally, iodine deficiency is responsible for a 10-15 Intelligence Quotient (IQ) unit loss in the population. This is because iodine is the basic element needed for thyroid hormone composition, and thyroid hormone is crucial in the early development process of the body, particularly the brain. During pregnancy, iodine deficiency can affect the motor and cognitive development of the children.

Vitamin D

Less than 10% of vitamin D is obtained from dietary sources, while the rest is mainly from exposure to ultraviolet radiation. Researchers have found that there is a correlation between the vitamin D status of the mother in the early pregnancy stage and delayed neurocognitive development.

Vitamin B12

This vitamin plays a major role in brain function and development. Deficiency in this vitamin might lead to pernicious anemia, which affects cognitive development, and a lack of B12 vitamins can lead to irreversible brain damage.

The Aging Brain

Just like every other part of the body, the brain ages as time flies. The structure and metabolic pathways in the brain get altered gradually with age. That is, there is a decline in the brain volume in the white and grey matter of the brain. With aging comes the development of amyloid plaques, an increase in white matter lesions, Lewy bodies, synaptic dystrophy, neurofibrillary tangles, and neuron loss. All these are implied to cause cognitive decline. Consequently, cognitive function declines with age, and it has been estimated by scientists that billions of people aged 60 years or above are projected to be affected by dementia and depression by 2050. Also, serotonin and dopamine decline up to about 10% per decade from the beginning of adulthood.

During the aging process, most changes in cognitive function are observed in the memory. Mild Cognitive Impairment (MCI) is a medical condition whereby the affected people have shown some pieces of evidence of cognitive impairment but do not meet the requirement for the diagnosis of dementia. The most popular kind of dementia is Alzheimer's disease, and it accounts for about 62% of most cases. Also, depression in the aging population is often referred to as late-life depression, which is more commonly found in females than males.

Neurotransmitters

Neurotransmitters are brain chemicals that allow effective communication throughout the brain and the body. They affect concentration, mood, sleep, carbohydrate cravings, addictions, and weight. When the neurotransmitters are not balanced, they can lead to anxiety, insomnia, pain, and depression. There are five important neurotransmitters: serotonin, dopamine, acetylcholine, Gamma-aminobutyric (GABA), and norepinephrine, and they are all required for alertness, learning, memory, and sleep.

According to researchers, neurotransmitters are directly linked to our diet. Certain foods will increase good neurotransmitters, while others will increase one's risks of cognitive problems, stress, and allergies.

Food affects how neurotransmitters are made in the gut and how it also affects the mind and brain. Also, scientists have found a correlation between friendly bacteria and the production of GABA, which exhibits the complex relationship between the gut and the brain.

Serotonin

Serotonin plays a major role in brain activities. It aids memory and learning. A low level of serotonin can lead to headaches, disorders, and depression. Foods like bananas, walnuts, kiwis, and eggs help to increase serotonin levels and make one happier, energized, and less foggy.

Dopamine

Dopamine controls and regulates the brain's pleasure and reward centers. High amounts of dopamine improve attention, memory, learning, mood, movement, and sleep. Abnormal levels of dopamine may cause schizophrenia and Parkinson's disease. Foods like Spirulina and eggs will help to improve attention span, memory, and mood.

Acetylcholine

Acetylcholine is built from the basic compound chlorine, which is a vital precursor for acetylcholine. So, foods rich in choline must Brussels sprouts and egg yolks can be eaten to raise acetylcholine levels.

GABA

Gaba sends information to several parts of the body and helps to reduce anxiety, provide a sense of calmness, and improve sleep. GABA is a by-product of microorganisms and plants; it can only be found in fermented foods.

Norepinephrine

Norepinephrine is primarily responsible for that "fight or flight" reaction you may have in stressful situations. It affects attention, mood, and motivation. Foods like avocados, pumpkin seeds, almonds, and lima beans will help to increase your norepinephrine levels.

Foods that Can Help Your Neurotransmitters

- Sesame seeds
- Raw pumpkin seeds
- Sunflower seeds
- Bananas
- Raw-dried dates
- Oats
- Spirulina
- Raw almonds
- Raw spinach
- Watercress
- Millet
- Pumpkin leaves
- Cacao
- Buckwheat
- Horseradish
- Turnip greens

Chapter Four

The Gut

The gastrointestinal (GI) tract is very crucial to human health. It helps in the transportation of food from the mouth to the stomach, the conversion of the food into absorbable nutrients, which are stored as energy, and the excretion of waste out of the body. Over the years, scientists have discovered that the GI tract performs a more complex job than it was previously known for. Most people assume that the gut is the stomach, but that is not the case. The stomach is part of the GI, while the gut is the entire GI from the mouth to the anus. Therefore, the gut is the pathway from your mouth to your anus. The human body contains more bacteria than human cells. These bacteria are called the microbiome. Most of the bacteria present in our body reside in the gut, and they are also referred to as gut microbiota or gut flora. The bacteria in our body are said to play several roles in our overall health. A healthy gut consists of a diversity of bacteria that maintains wellness. Gut health is the function and balance of everything that happens in the gut. A healthy gut promotes good physical and mental health. The human gut microbiome can be found in the gut, and it is a collection of microbiota that is an incredibly complex ecosystem of archaea, fungi, viruses, and bacteria.

Our gut microbiome is unique to each individual and can be influenced by humans through;

- Medication (acid suppressants, antibiotics, etc.).
- Feeding methods (artificial milk, breast milk, solid foods).
- Dietary habits.
- The way foods are cooked.
- Weight gain.
- Environmental factors and lifestyle (rural vs. urban locations, exercise).

While the activities above can help influence the gut microbiome, there are some factors that humans cannot influence, and they include;

- Aging
- Genetics
- Delivery mode (vaginal delivery vs. C-section)
- Gestational age (preterm birth vs. full-term birth)
- Anatomical part of the GI (the large intestine contains a higher diversity of gut microbiome than the small intestine).

What Constitutes a Healthy Gut Microbiome?

- The richness of the gut microbial; the amount of microbial genes in the hut is an indicator of good metabolic and overall health.
- Diversity; the amount of different species in a specific habitat is a hallmark of good gut health.
- Resilience, resistance, and stability over time; the ability of the gut microbiota to resist perturbation (e.g., imbalanced diet).

Several ailments, such as diabetes, obesity, allergies, cancer, digestive ailments, and neurodegenerative diseases, have been associated with gut microbiota imbalance.

Microbes existed before humans arrived, and the intestine is one of the most densely populated microbial habitats on earth. The human skin, nose, mouth and throat, lungs, and vagina also house microbes.

Importance of the gut microbiota

Nutrition

- It helps to digest certain foods like fiber which humans are not able to digest.
- It helps to produce important molecules that benefit the body.
- It synthesizes some essential vitamins like vitamin K and amino acids.
- It facilitates the absorption of dietary minerals like calcium, iron, and magnesium.

Defense

- It degrades toxic compounds.
- It trains the immune system to differentiate between harmful and not harmful substances.
- It fights harmful microorganisms.

Behavior

- It influences our moods and behaviors.

The delivery mode of a child influences the gut microbiota in early life. An infant born vaginally is colonized by the mother's gut and vaginal microbiota first. However, a baby delivered through cesarean section (C-Section) is exposed to the skin and hospital environment microbiota first. So, a baby born vaginally obtains the bacteria resembling the mother's, which shows a low level of diversity. Over time, the mode of feeding also impacts the infant's microbiota. Human breast milk contains live bacteria and a variety of complex carbohydrates that babies cannot digest. These complex carbohydrates act as prebiotics that influence the infant's gut. However, formula-fed infants develop a microbiota that resembles that of an adult and have a higher overall bacteria diversity. Solid foods and fiber also increase gut bacteria diversity.

The gut microbiota changes with time from infancy to old age. It is highly variable in newborns, and it tends to be relatively stable as they age and is accompanied by a lower level of diversity and loss of vital genes that produce short-chain fatty acids. Age-related changes in the gut microbiomes can be partly avoidable through lifestyle. This means that when you take care of your gut, it improves the overall health of the gut.

Western Diet and Western Microbiome

There is a significant difference between the microbiome of children in Europe and Africa. The Western microbiome lacks diversity and has a lot more bacteria from the group Firmicutes than from the group Bacteroidetes. Firmicutes and Bacteroidetes are the two types of bacteria that dominate the gut's ecology. Firmicutes assist the body in extracting more calories from food and help absorb fats. Firmicutes are linked with weight gain when they dominate the gut's ecology. However, Bacteroidetes do not have this ability. Therefore, a higher level of Firmicutes and a lower level of Bacteroidetes are linked to a higher risk of obesity. It is more common in people in urban areas than in rural areas.

There is a link between gut bacteria and being overweight and obese. People who are obese and overweight have their gut microbiota showing signs of dysbiosis, unlike people who keep a healthy weight. Dysbiosis can also result from consuming antibiotics, irregular eating habits, consuming sugary and fatty foods, too much alcohol, and chronic stress.

Being overweight and obese is a result of excess body fat. Genetics favored body fat many years ago when most people were malnourished. Genetics favored fat storage with technological advancement, economic boom, and sustainability. The Body Mass Index (BMI) is a calculation that shows the difference between overweight and obese persons. The BMI estimates healthy body weight and actual body fat percentage, which can be determined by muscle mass and waist circumference. Most athletes have a higher BMI because they have more muscle mass than non-athletes. BMI is calculated using a person's height and weight.

The formula is: **BMI $= \mathbf{kg/m^2}$** (kg is a person's weight in kilograms and m^2 is their height in meters squared)

The healthy range is between 18.5 and 24.9. A BMI of 25.0 or more is overweight. Too much fat in the body can lead to many problems like lethargy, knee and back pain, heart-related problems, high cholesterol, depression, PCOS, and body image issues.

A large intestine is a safe place for trillions of mutually beneficial microbes that make up your gut microbiota. The gut bacteria form an ecosystem vital for metabolism, hunger, and digestion. Exercise, a balanced diet, and emotional well-being are crucial for healthy, diversified gut bacteria. Bacteria like Christensenella minuta, Akkermansia muciniphila, and Lactobacillus gasseri play a vital role in weight loss, and prebiotics can help increase their numbers in the gut. Natural prebiotics can be taken to fuel skinny bacteria. They include rhubarb extract, garlic, bamboo shoots, flaxseeds, potato starch, cranberries, and black tea. Weight loss bacteria do not exist, but certain foods can be eaten to prevent weight gain. These foods help to multiply the microbiomes, which leads to higher metabolism.

Gastric acidity plays a vital role in the gut. It helps to shape the composition and diversity of the microbial community. It is important to note that the production of a cycle of excessive bile acid from the liver to break down fats can be why the body is in an acidic state.

Hyperacidity (acid reflux or gastritis) occurs when there is inflammation of the stomach lining due to a person's lifestyle, like excessive alcohol consumption. Other problems include depression, weight gain, frustration, and colon ulcers. Common symptoms of an acidic body are emotional discomfort, build-up of stress, abdominal cramps, bloating, stomach ulcers, heartburn, and acid reflux. Also, it will be difficult to lose weight in an acidic body.

The nutrients and calories are extracted and metabolized based on the foods we consume. This process leaves behind an ash residue. So, when a portion of acidic food is eaten, the ash displays high acidic levels. The quantity of ash left behind by a particular food consumed determines the pH of the food, grouping it into either acid-forming or alkalizing food.

Some Highly Acidic Food to Avoid

Caffeinated Sodas- Caffeinated sodas are acidic, whether they are sugary or sugar-free. Even though tea, coffee, and other caffeinated beverages boost energy, they can also lead to rebound fatigue after the effect wears off and leaves you craving more soda.

Hydrogenated Fats- Manufacturers make liquid vegetables creamier, converting unsaturated fats into saturated fats through hydrogenation. This process is very dangerous to the body and can affect the heart and increase a person's risk of cancer. Foods like fried snacks like chips, doughnuts, cookies, and crackers should be avoided or eaten in small quantities.

Processed and Stale Foods- Foods like packaged foods, pizzas, meat, and cereals are highly acidic.

Milk- This largely depends on the dairy farm you get your milk from. Are they fed soya, corn silage, or grain with hormone injections? Or are they given access to pasture, or are they grass-fed?

Gluten and GMOs- Soya, wheat, and corn should be avoided so that the acidic level can be minimized because they harm the kidneys and liver.

Acidity and alkalinity in the fluids and tissues of humans range from 0 to 14 when measured. The human body maintains a regulated pH level. A normal pH level of 7 is neutral, more than 7 is alkaline, and less than 7 is acidic. The kidney controls the body's pH. The kidney does this by excreting and absorbing acid and alkaline ions from urine and the body. Alkaline diets help lower inflammation in the stomach, which aids digestion and prevents acid reflux acid. Alkalinity has many benefits, such as decreasing chronic pain reducing chronic pain, keeping gut microbes in symbiosis, and balancing hormones.

How to Keep Your Alkalinity in Check

1. Sit upright or take a slow walk after meals. This will help break down food in the stomach and lower the risk of indigestion and acid reflux.

2. Avoid eating dinner late at night. Early dinner is best because it makes it possible for your body system to reboot until next noon.

3. Limit caffeine intake, and lean towards berry smoothies and herbal potions. Starting your day with a berry smoothie and banana has positive benefits on the body because fruits are alkaline and antioxidant. Coconut water is also good because it is alkaline and promotes vitality and longevity, unlike caffeine.

4. Avoid GMOs, gluten, and fast foods. Go vegan! Opt for almond, rice, coconut, and hemp or seed milk instead of regular milk. Avoid pasta, wraps, gluten-rich bread, corn, MSG, and fried fast foods.

5. Go to bed at night with a free-flowing cloth. Do not sleep in tight and ill-fitting clothes. This is because the tightness can lead to stomach distention and a backward flow of food content.

6. Drinking enough water will help balance the pH levels in the body. It will eject excess acidic ions from the kidney and keep the cells hydrated and more alkaline.

7. Consume more brain foods like unsaturated fatty acids because they lower inflammation and increase the number of good microbes.

Hormones and the Gut

The gut microbes play a vital role here. They help to absorb and release all nutrients into the bloodstream to nourish all nine glands. Therefore, this helps the glands to work as a team, from growth, sleep, and sexual drive to metabolism. Serotonin and dopamine are important hormones produced in the gut, and the activity of the glands depends on gut health.

The balance of hormones has an effect and is also affected by all the systems in the body. An emerging field in science called integrative nutrition centers on the underlying workings of the gut, and the physical and mental causes of illness, rather than just treating the symptoms.

So, what is a hormone? A hormone is a chemical that contains specialist cells, often within the endocrine glands. These hormones are released into the bloodstream to communicate or send messages to other body parts. These chemical messengers are present in all multicellular organisms and provide an internal communication system between cells found in distant parts of the body.

Major Female Hormones

- Estrogen
- Progesterone
- Cortisol
- Thyroid

Major Male Hormones

- Pregnenolone
- Testosterone
- DHEA
- Androstenedione

There is a group of endocrine glands that help produce hormones used as chemical messengers throughout the body to regulate significant processes like metabolism, growth, reproduction, and sleep. Gamma-aminobutyric acid (GABA) is a vital chemical messenger that contributes to vision, motor control, and other cortical functions. GABA also helps to control our fear and anxiety. The hormones produced by the glands are emitted into the bloodstream. They bind to a particular receptor cell to do its assigned tasks.

Extremely low or high thyroid function is related to your metabolism, microbiome, diet, sleep, emotional stress, lifestyle, inflammation, and exercise. It is not due to genetics. The hormones released by the thyroid, insulin, and cortisol are the 'big three' that control metabolism and weight. The pituitary gland produces and releases the hormone. It controls the production of thyroid hormones, thyroxine, and triiodothyronine which are responsible for maintaining the body's metabolic rate, digestive function, muscle control, and heart and brain development.

A hyperpermeable gut makes it possible for pathogens to attack the thyroid gland, leading to an autoimmune condition such as low or high thyroid functioning. The common thyroid disorders are Hashimoto's disease, thyroid cancer, hypothyroidism, Grave's disease, goiter, hyperthyroidism, and thyroid nodules. Symptoms of a malfunctioning thyroid include constipation, numbness in the hands, fatigue, tingling, change in body temperature, water retention, excessive weight gain, excessive weight loss, depression, water retention, hair fall, muscle and joint ache, brain fog, and longer menstrual cycles.

Also, the gut microbiota improves the lives of those living with type 2 diabetes. The gut helps to break down food rich in polyphenols into metabolites. People with type 2 diabetes cannot produce adequate insulin because their beta cells no longer work properly. Therefore, the gut microbiota needs to be fed well in other to produce enough insulin and improve the blood-glucose level. Diabetes is a severe medical condition in which sugar level builds up in the bloodstream. Insulin helps remove the sugar or glucose from the blood and into your cells so your body can use it for energy. Type 2 diabetes causes the body cells not to respond adequately to insulin and causes the body not to produce enough insulin. Some early diabetes symptoms include lack of energy, constant hunger, frequent urination, itchy skin, weight gain, irritability, dry mouth, and fatigue. Chronic symptoms include slow healing of cuts or sores, dark, patchy skin, depression, yeast infection, and foot pain.

Chapter Five

————— · · ● · · —————

The Immune System

The immune system was discovered basically because of the need to prevent the spread of disease and develop better treatments for sicknesses. Many years ago, scientists wanted to vaccinate people against infections, which led to vaccines being developed to fight the diseases. These vaccines were developed before anyone could prove that microbes were the cause of illnesses or that the immune cells could kill microbes.

The immune system is a network of cells, tissues, and organs that work as a team to protect the body against the attacks of foreign intruders. These intruders are germs or microbes, which are minute, infection-causing organisms like viruses, bacteria, fungi, and parasites. These microbes can enter the body because the human body provides a perfect environment for many microbes to gain entrance into the body. The immune system helps to keep them from entering the body, and if they enter, it seeks them out and destroys them. If the immune system is crippled or hits the wrong target, a rush of diseases like allergies, AIDS, or arthritis could be unleashed.

The immune system is a mechanism that allows a person to differentiate between 'self' and 'non-self.' A healthy immune system can distinguish between the body's cells and a foreign cell. This means that the immune system is linked to our health, and every disease is tied to it.

Weak and Overactive Immune System

A broken-down immune system opens the door to deadly infections. Infections are just but one disease. Other sicknesses like cancer can happen because the immune system has been weakened, and the immune system cannot detect the cancer cells. Anything that sets off the immune response is referred to as an antigen. An antigen is a microbe. Also, cells or tissues from some other person except an identical twin can act as an antigen and carry a non-self-maker, and the tissue or cell will be rejected. Abnormal cases could also spring up when the immune system mistakes itself for non-self and initiates an attack against the body's tissues or cells. When this happens, this occurrence is called autoimmune disease. Examples of this include arthritis and diabetes. In other situations, the immune system reacts to a harmless foreign substance like ragweed pollen. This results in an allergy which is an antigen called an allergen.

The opposite of a weak immune system is an overactive system, and an overactive immune system leads to autoimmune diseases, which occur when the immune system becomes active at the wrong time and in the wrong place. An example of an autoimmune disease is Lupus erythematosus, a collection of autoimmune diseases whereby antibodies initiate attacks on several organs in the body like the heart, lungs, kidneys, brain, joints, and spinal cords. An overactive immunity can cause severe inflammation. For example, asthmatic patients have a trigger-happy-immune system that causes chronic lung inflammation when exposed to several environmental factors. People living with psoriasis have chronic inflammation of the skin and joints. Those with Crohn's disease and ulcerative colitis have severe gut inflammation, which causes bloating, abdominal pain, and intestinal bleeding. If there is no treatment for ulcerative colitis, persistent inflammation can cause colon cancer. If you like to get more information about inflammation, I can recommend "THE COMPLETE ANTI-INFLAMMATORY

DIET FOR BEGINNER: Ultimate Guide to Restoring Your Immune System, Healing Inflammation, and Reversing Disease", written by Emma Collins. She covers every aspect of inflammation in this book very readable way.

The Immune System and the Brain

Studies have found that the immune system consists of idiosyncratic, self-regulatory properties and functions like the endocrine and nervous systems. In addition, the immune system responds to stimuli; it can be compared to an extra sensory organ.

Two pathways link the brain and the immune system. They include the autonomic nervous system and the neuroendocrine outflow through the pituitary. These pathways deliver biologically active molecules that are capable of interacting with the cells and immune system. The primary and secondary lymphoid organs are stimulated with noradrenergic postganglionic sympathetic nerve fibers. The peptidergic nerve fibers are also in the thymus, bone marrow, spleen, lymph nodes, and mucosal-associated lymphoid tissue.

Furthermore, the nerve fibers form proximate neuroeffector junctions with macrophages and lymphocytes. The neurotransmitters emitted from these nerves spread out to act in distant places, which further extends the potential for neural-immune interactions. Likewise, the lymphocytes, monocytes/macrophages, and granulocytes own the receptors for the neurotransmitters.

Gut and Immunity

The gut is the first line of defense of the body because it contains varying strains and bacterial warriors that fight against illnesses and build immunity. So, most of our immunity can be found in the gut. The gut flora uses the colon (which is covered with a mucus layer) as food to grow and multiply. The digestive system from the mouth to the anus is also the first line of defense for other organs like the brain, heart, lungs, and kidneys. The microbes defend the body against bad bacteria from inside and outside the body. There are some cells in the lining of the gut that excrete huge amounts of antibodies into the gut. Over ninety percent of the healthy gut microbiome leads the microbial ecosystem from the GI tract. The gut microbiome is a dynamic central regulator of mitochondrial function in intestinal cells, which consists of immune and epithelial cells. When the immune system is under a virus attack, the gut microbiota sends signals to the mitochondrial mucosal cells (the body's main power).

The gut microbiome is very active in interacting and shaping the host mucosal immune system and regulating intestinal homeostasis. This leads to stability in equilibrium between interdependent elements. Microbiotic signaling developed in the immune cells eradicates invading viruses and pathogens and the production of millions of cytokines. Cytokine is a category of proteins, peptides, and glycoproteins that are secreted by particular cells of the immune system. Microbes are responsible for signaling the cells and molecules tha help mediate and regulate immunity and inflammation to protect the body from any attack. Then the microbiota in the gut signals the mitochondrion to get ready for battle.

The Mental Sickness

Sometimes falling sick could be more mental than physical. It can come in various forms, like feeling anxious about your health and googling symptoms to know what exactly is wrong with you because you think you are sick. Sometimes, the fear of falling ill is in itself a form of illness. This could be psychosomatic. This behavior is also known as nosophobia, hypochondriasis, or illness anxiety disorder. Many people develop illnesses in their minds and start believing that they have that specific illness.

There is always that one person who is always negative and usually thinks they are sick. Such people have wild imaginations, and they always imagine the worst-case scenario. There is power in the mind, and constant fear of falling sick can make you feel unwell. Having a good and healthy immune system also involves being emotionally stable and happy. A positive state of mind can also act like a potent medicine that protects one from sicknesses and boosts immunity. Mental wellness is a very significant aspect of your overall health. Mental wellness contributes to healing, making decisions, and boosting immunity. So, having a healthy gut and a positive mindset work simultaneously. Therefore, your immunity depends on your physical, mental, and emotional balance.

Boosting Immunity Emotionally and Mentally

Avoid Negativity- Do not indulge in negative conversations. Speaking negatively impacts your mental health and can affect your overall body and well-being. Only entertain positive conversations.

Enhance your Productivity- Having an aimless day will affect your productivity levels and your physical and mental well-being. Set daily targets and goals and stick to them because you get happy when you achieve your daily goals.

Rigid Mindset about Medicines- Medicines are not the only way you can get healed from sicknesses. Sometimes having a positive mindset toward life can go a long way. Change your rigid mindsets about medicines and listen to your gut feelings. Meditation helps calm the body and allows the body to heal naturally.

Avoid Negative News- Negative news is not good, so try to avoid negative or bad news that can affect your mood and mental health. It is best to avoid negative news because it can become addictive. You can do this by trying out digital cleansing and detox.

Avoid Negative Labels and Statements- Negative labels and statements will have adverse effects on you mentally. Have a positive attitude towards life, and do not label yourself negatively. Do not call yourself names like 'worthless,' 'not good enough,' ugly,' etc.

Breathing Rate- Watch how you breathe, and avoid stressful situations that drain your energy. Try deep breathing. It helps to reduce stress, increase dopamine, and boost immunity.

Foods that Boost the Immune System

Mushrooms- Edible mushrooms like the white button mushroom are a good source of bioactive, including beta-glucan, an immune-stimulating dietary fiber. Studies have found that eating mushrooms activates the gut, which stimulates the immune system to produce antibodies. The antibodies will be spread to the mucous membranes, where they will be discharged in the saliva. Other studies involving shiitake, enoki, maitake, oyster, and chanterelle mushrooms showed that the mushrooms activated the immune defenses.

Broccoli Sprouts- Broccoli sprouts are three-day plant tendrils that have a mild, nutty taste. Broccoli contains sulforaphane which is a powerful bioactive. Broccoli sprouts contain up to one hundred times more sulforaphane than regular full-grown broccoli. It would be best if you chewed your broccoli sprouts thoroughly because chewing breaks the plant cell walls to emit an enzyme called myrosinase. This vital enzyme converts inactive sulforaphane into an active form in your mouth.

Aged Garlic- Garlic is seen as a food ingredient as well as a health remedy. Aged garlic remains nearly odor-free, unlike fresh garlic, which has a strong, pungent smell. Aged garlic can be used as a dietary supplement because it retains potent bioactives like apigenin which can affect the immune system.

Extra Virgin Olive Oil- Extra virgin olive oil is a component of the Mediterranean diet, and it contains bioactive like oleocanthal, oleic acid, and hydroxytyrosol, which improves the immune system. Studies have revealed that olive oil lowers the body's reaction to allergens. Additionally, the hydroxytyrosol bioactive found in the oil helps to produce interleukin-10, which soothes and calms inflammation. Also, it is important to note that not all oils contain the same level of hydroxytyrosol.

Ellagic Acid- Ellagic acid is a potent bioactive consisting of health defense activating properties, and it is found in most popular foods. Foods with the highest amounts of ellagic acid include chestnuts, walnuts, blackberries, raspberries, and pomegranate. Ellagic acid has antiangiogenic effects, which are known to starve tumors and prevent their growth. This acid also helps locate and track cancer cells and destroy them.

Vitamin C- Citrus fruits like oranges, tangerines, pomelos, grapefruits, lemons, and lime produce white blood cells in the body because they are rich in vitamin C.

Flaxseeds - Flaxseeds play a vital role in emptying the bowels. Both brown and golden flax seeds have rich nutrients like dietary fiber and omega-3 fats. Flaxseeds are good for the heart and gut. Also, it has plant compounds called lignans, which have antioxidant properties. They help to lower blood pressure and improve cholesterol levels.

Cruciferous Vegetables- These vegetables contain phytochemicals that fight cancer. Some leafy greens include spinach, cabbage, brussels sprouts, garden cress, bok choy, and broccoli which improve immunity.

Tumeric (Haldi)- Tumeric can be used for cooking and many other things. It is a spice used as a nutritional supplement and provides several benefits for the body and brain. Its benefits stem from its main ingredient, curcumin. Tumeric contains bioactive and natural anti-inflammatory compounds that help fight invaders and repair damaged bodies. Studies have shown that it helps fight heart disease, cancer, metabolic syndrome, Alzheimer's disease, and other degenerative conditions.

Coconut Oil- This oil consists of medium-chain triglycerides, which help lower cholesterol levels and other fats in the body. Taking a tablespoon of cold-pressed coconut oil on an empty stomach benefits the gut. It helps to seal the gut and prevent brain leakiness.

Caraway Seeds- These seeds are very beneficial for the digestive system. Caraway seeds help to relieve nausea, cramps, and bloating. They also help to release gas from the body.

The Gut and Hunger

Certain hormone-producing microbes send signals to you when you have reached a point of satiety or not and communicate the same to the brain. Leptin and ghrelin help stimulate and suppress hunger and satiety to maintain optimal weight and energy.

Some people are always hungry, which can be due to a lack of knowledge about food choices or nutrition, emotional trauma, dehydration, stressful lifestyle, acidity, thyroid, diabetes, and depression. It could also be due to eating a diet lacking protein, fats, fiber, etc.

Tips to Help You Feel Full

1. Revamp your fridge. Instead of storing junk like pizza, etc., replace them with fruits, yogurts, water, and vegetables.

2. Eating always can make you produce more of the hormone insulin, so eat whole foods so that your hours between meals will be increased. Examples include yogurt, rice, legumes, salad, nut butter, and apples. Avoid eating simple carbs like wafers and biscuits.

3. Have more high-fiber, low-calorie foods like green vegetables, whole grains, monosaturated fats, and protein.

4. Be hydrated with water and not sodas. Most people mistake thirst for hunger; always keep a bottle of water with you to avoid taking sodas.

5. Get adequate sleep.

6. Mediation, laughter, and exercise should be used to take care of emotional/stress eating.

Prebiotics and Probiotics

Prebiotics and probiotics are very important when considering nutrition because they are more than capable of preventing sicknesses and illnesses. They play both different and complementary roles in gut health. What are prebiotics? Prebiotics are living organisms and substances that come from some types of carbohydrates (mostly fibers) that humans cannot digest. Therefore, they are food for bacteria in the gut. The good bacteria in your gut depend on this fiber for food and multiplication. They help to fight bacteria like E. coli and salmonella.

On the other hand, probiotics are living organisms that live off of the benefits of the host. For example, when milk is fermented with lactic acid, bacteria multiply the nourishing and beneficial bacteria in it and boost health. These foods can be found in some supplements and foods.

The good bacteria in the body help defend the body against disease-causing bacteria, balance hormones, strengthen the immune system, improve brain function, and repress uncontrollable inflammation.

How to Get Prebiotics into Your System

Prebiotics are the dietary fiber that feeds the friendly bacteria in your gut. They help the microbiome to produce nutrients for the colon cells, which leads to a healthier digestive system. These nutrients include short-chain fatty acids like acetate, butyrate, and propionate. Below are some healthy ways to get prebiotics into your system;

- *Leeks-* belong to the same family as garlic and onions. They contain insulin fiber which promotes gut bacteria and helps break down fat.

- **Garlic-** an herb that acts as a prebiotic that promotes the growth of beneficial Bifidobacteria in the gut, which prevents disease-promoting bacteria from growing.
- **Onions-** onions strengthen the gut flora, which breaks down fat and improves the immune system. Onions also have antibiotic properties and are healthy.
- **Apple-** helps to decrease bad bacteria and increase butyrate. They also have anti-inflammatory properties and help with digestion.
- **Flaxseed-** contains soluble fiber from mucilage gums and insoluble fiber from lignin and cellulose, which is very good for gut bacteria.
- **Dandelion greens-** are a good source of fiber and can be used as a salad filler. The insulin in dandelions helps decrease constipation and improve the immune system.
- **Raw Chicory root-** raw chicory root is high in insulin and is a prebiotic fiber that aids digestion and prevents constipation.
- **Bananas-** bananas are rich in fiber, vitamins, and minerals. Also, resistant starch in green, unripe bananas contains high prebiotic levels.
- **Oats-** oats are healthy grains rich in prebiotics benefits, resistant starch, and beta-glucan fiber, which lowers LDL cholesterol, controls sugar, and lowers cancer risks.

- **Herbs-** some herbs are also good sources of prebiotics, like burdock dandelion root, and Triphala.
- **Chickpea-** chickpea is rich in fiber, iron, and B vitamins. Also, it can be used in patties, salads, or as hummus.
- **Lentils-** lentils stimulate good bacteria and aid digestion. It does not matter if it is red or pink. It is very beneficial to the body.
- **Asparagus-** asparagus is a very good source of prebiotics, and it helps the gut bacteria.

Probiotics

Probiotics are derived from the Latin word 'pro,' which means 'for,' and 'biotic,' which means 'life.' This means that probiotics help to create an environment in the gut for good bacteria to thrive and bad bacteria to be suppressed.

Types of Probiotics

1. **Lactobacilli-** lactobacilli produce lactase, an enzyme that breaks down lactose, the sugar present in milk. Lactobacilli help in the fermentation of carbohydrates in the gut, which produces lactic acid. Lactic acid is crucial because it helps to

create an acidic environment in the digestive tract and prevents many harmful microorganisms. It helps to increase the absorption of minerals like copper, magnesium, calcium, and iron.

2. ***Bifidobacteria-*** this type of bacteria can be found within the mucus lining of the large intestine and the vaginal tract. Bifidobacteria stop disease-causing bacteria and yeast, control acidity and alkalinity levels protect against bad bacteria, and increase the absorption of magnesium, calcium, iron, and zinc.

Probiotics not only have benefits for the gut but also help treat and prevent many common illnesses like arthritis, high blood pressure, allergies, gastrointestinal issues, acidity, cancer, depression, anxiety, etc. It is very easy to get probiotics into your body naturally and by taking supplements.

Advantages of Consuming Probiotics

- It improves mood.
- It boosts immunity.
- It lowers blood pressure.
- It lowers cholesterol.
- It cures urinary tract infections.
- It improves sex drive.

- It improves oral hygiene.

- It enhances memory and learning.

- It aids digestion.

- It balances hormones.

- It balances blood sugar levels.

- It slows the rate of absorption of dietary fats. Therefore, it helps in weight loss.

- It prevents heart disease by reducing inflammation.

- It prevents eczema and allergies.

Foods that Contain Probiotics

- Yogurt

- Green vegetable juice

- Beetroot.

- Aged cheese

- Naturally fermented raw unpasteurized cider vinegar.

Chapter Six

Leaky Gut

A leaky gut (intestinal permeability of the gut barrier) is a problem that occurs when the small intestine lining has been damaged, and the gaps in the intestinal walls begin to loosen. When this happens, it becomes easier for larger and foreign substances like undigested food particles and toxins to leak into the bloodstream. This can lead to an autoimmune response in the body, including allergic and inflammatory reactions such as eczema, IBS, thyroid, and migraine.

Everything is left unguarded when the gates of the gut and villi open up, causing hyperpermeability. The villi only allow micronutrients to pass through so the cells and organs will be nourished. Zonulin released by the gut cells helps to regulate the tight junction structure and function, which strongly holds and guards the wall. Higher levels of zonulin lead to a breakdown of tight junctions between intestinal epithelial cells, which increases porousness. Studies have shown that an elevated level of zonulin leads to several autoimmune, neoplastic diseases, type 1 diabetes, inflammatory, asthma, juvenile non-alcoholic fatty liver, inflammatory bowel disease, multiple sclerosis, and rheumatoid arthritis.

Foreign substances attach themselves to healthy cells or organs when they seep through the gaps in the intestinal walls and into the bloodstream. This causes a flare-up and inflammation of the immune system and, eventually, the entire body. It compromises your immune system and white blood cells, which protect your body from diseases, infections, and foreign bodies. When these toxins and pathogens remain attached to your healthy cells, they remain afloat in your blood and cause damage to your gut.

The gut lining of the intestinal permeability can be likened to a filter (muslin cheesecloth) which holds food back and allows the right nutrients to pass through it. Also, autoimmune diseases cause a leaky gut. Here, the cells fight against each other, mistaking each other as enemies.

The Leaky Gut Syndrome

A syndrome is a combination of problems, signs, and symptoms of medical and mental conditions; a leaky gut syndrome can lead to moodiness and depression. In the body, there is an extensive intestinal lining that covers a huge surface that has a hundred trillion microbiomes. And when they are imbalanced, you may have a leaky gut.

Some Factors which can cause Leaky Gut

- Eating packaged and fast foods.
- Generally, stress is not good for the body, and chronic stress can lead to many gastrointestinal disorders, such as a leaky gut.
- Severe inflammation from a bad lifestyle and stress can sometimes be passed from mother to child and lead to a leaky gut.
- Not drinking enough water can dehydrate your cells and organs, and this can cause bile to become more concentrated, which leads to acidity, constipation, microbial imbalances, and inflammation.
- Consuming too much sugar like bagels, waffles, desserts, and kulfis. This can increase the number of harmful substances in the body, which can cause a leaky gut.

- Suppose you suffer from acid reflux, acidity, stomach burn, or heartburn. In that case, there is a probability that there is an excess secretion of acids in the gastric glands in the stomach. Stomach ache, gas, and bad breath are common signs of a leaky gut.
- Consuming aerated beverages such as acid bombs can lead to acidity. This is because aerated beverages contain excess artificial sweeteners.
- Consuming excessive glutens can lead to a leaky gut. They can be found in wheat, processed fast foods, and bread.
- Consuming antacids, antibiotics, and other medicines can lead to a leaky gut. Acid blockers only suppress the acid coming up the food pipe, and the acid remains in the body. This impedes the absorption of essential nutrients like calcium, zinc, and vitamin B12.
- Excessive exposure to screen time can indirectly lead to a leaky gut. This is because cell phones emit radio frequency which may lead to a microbiome imbalance and even cancer. Excessive screen time can disturb your sleep patterns and ruin the body's circadian rhythm.
- Yeast is naturally present in the body, and an imbalanced diet can feed the wrong microbiomes and lead to an overgrowth of yeast. Thrush, candidiasis, and diapers are common fungal

infections, and when left untreated, they can lead to a leaky gut.

Some Symptoms of a Leaky Gut

- Overnight bloating
- Constipation
- Digestive problems
- Obesity
- Stomach cramps and diarrhea
- Diabetes
- Autoimmune diseases
- Migraine
- Cancer
- Dementia
- Common cold, cough, or flu
- Autism
- Widespread inflammation
- Alzheimer's disease
- Low immunity
- Throbbing headaches
- Parkinson's disease
- Eczema
- PCOS

- Thyroid
- Lupus
- Asthma attacks
- Unbearable PMS
- Crohn's disease
- Skin allergies like pimples and acne
- Food allergies and intolerances
- Celiac disease
- Depression
- Rheumatoid arthritis
- Difficulty in concentration
- Hashimoto's disease
- Anxiety
- Suicidal thoughts
- Erratic mood swings
- Difficulty in concentration
- ADD
- ADHD
- Addictions
- Frequent pill popping to feel better
- Sugar and salty food cravings

Sugar and Gluten

The major factors which affect the gut are sugar and gluten. Most foods consumed today are unnatural and extremely high in sugar and gluten. Foods that are high in sugar are associated with overweight and obesity, which are risk factors for diabetes. Studies have discovered a strong link between obesity and death. Sugar is addictive, and bad bacteria in the gut love addiction. An imbalance in your microbiome causes you to become an addict.

Ways in which Sugar Affects the Body

- Sugar multiplies and causes an imbalance in your microbiome.
- Sugar quickens the aging and wrinkling process.
- Sugar causes glucose to spike and plunge.
- Sugar affects the cognitive fitness of the brain.
- Sugar accelerates the risk of obesity, gut leakiness, diabetes, and heart disease.

The term gluten is derived from the glue-like property of wet dough, which makes the dough elastic and soft, which makes bread rise when baking. It also makes bread chewy and satisfying. Gluten is a family of proteins obtained in foods like barley, wheat, rye, and spelt. The elastic nature of bread will not be made possible without gluten. Pizza dough will not be able to be thrown into the air without its stretchiness which allows it to land back on the hand without breaking. The two major proteins in the gluten of wheat are gliadin and glutenin. Gliadin is the cause of the majority of the adverse effects of gluten. Researchers have found that gliadin increases the Zonulin levels produced by your cells, leading to an increase in gut sensitivity, microbial imbalance, and permeability.

Gluten Intolerance or Sensitivity

When a gluten-sensitive person consumes too many gluten-rich processed products, their gut allows the passage of this protein which results in the inflammation of the entire body. The body becomes susceptible to wheat allergies, celiac, migraine, dermatitis, herpetiformis (DH), eczema, and other illnesses. Gluten sensitivity can also lead to acidity, bloating, stomach pain, fatigue, leaky gut, diarrhea, headache, celiac disease, constipation, gas, mood swings, drastic weight loss, digestive disorder (IBS), foul-smelling excreta, abdominal cramps, pain. A gluten-sensitive person can reverse gluten damage by staying away from gluten. A celiac patient can reduce the effects of the illness by eliminating gluten from the diet. Cereals, spelt, barley, rye, beer, bread, pizza, pasta, cookies, burger, and pastries are usually high in gluten.

A gluten-free diet involves eliminating all foods containing gluten. Most people make huge mistakes when they rely on ready-made and processed gluten-free pasta and cookies, which might be high in additives, calories, sugar, saturated fats, and sodium which are low in nutritional value. A good source of information about gluten is THE COMPLETE ANTI-INFLAMMATORY DIET FOR BEGINNERS, written by Emma Collins, which I already mentioned above in the inflammatory chapter.

Affordable and Available Gluten-Free Foods

Pay more attention to naturally gluten-free foods. They include garbanzo beans, pinto beans, lima beans, wild rice, brown rice, basmati rice, red rice, seeds, root vegetables, turnips, yams, sweet potatoes, and yellow potatoes. These foods have the required nutritious carbohydrate that is good for the body and is gluten-free. All fruits and vegetables are gluten-free and usually affordable at the store. You can always prepare your gluten-free snack like nuts, seeds, and dried fruit mixes, and all these are affordable. There are a lot of options available if you like baking. There are available gluten-free flours that you can use.

Leaky Brain

A leaky brain occurs when the blood-brain barrier (BBB) has been damaged. The brain has a semi-permeable diffusion barrier that prevents most compounds from entering the brain from the blood. When the tight junction gets broken or loose, the BBB becomes permeable, and toxins and harmful substances can enter the brain and cause damage, leading to inflammation. A leaky or inflamed brain can be the main cause of a simple migraine to Alzheimer's disease. Therefore, the link between the gut and the brain should not be underestimated and neglected because microbiomes live in the gut and can affect the brain positively and negatively.

Three cellular elements of the brain microvasculature compose the BBB. They include endothelial cells, astrocyte end-feet, and pericytes. The tight junctions in between the cerebral endothelial cells develop a diffusion barrier that selectively leaves out most blood-borne substances from getting into the brain. Any malfunctioning of the BBB, like the impairment of the tight junction seal, will lead to some neurologic diseases, such as strokes and inflammatory disorders. The major causes of the leaky brain are leaky gut, gut dysbiosis, autoimmune, chronic stress, dehydration, toxins, inflammation, obesity, poor choices of fats and high-calorie diets, obesity, liver damage, excessive sugar intake, erratic sleep patterns, vagus nerve dysfunction, processed and packages foods.

Signs that something might be wrong with your brain

- *Brain Fog-* Brain fog is a symptom of cognitive malfunction. It can cause mental fatigue or zoning out, poor concentration, and memory loss.
- *Headaches and migraines-* Persistent headaches and migraines could be good signs of inflammation of the brain.
- *Nausea and Vomiting-* Excess amounts of viruses and parasites in the body could be the reason why you might feel nauseous and sick every time.
- *Memory loss-* You should seek medical attention if you notice you lose your chain of thoughts often, lose items, or forget the names of those close to you.
- *Depression-* When you begin to fall into depression often, it could be a sign of problems with your brain.

Few things that can cause a leaky-gut brain

- *Packaged foods-* If you must buy packaged foods, read the packages well enough to know what is going into your body. Reading the contents written on the packages would let you know what foods to avoid. Avoid foods that are high in plain flour, preservatives, sugar, and sodium. All these are addictive and are engineered for overconsumption. Some of these foods have zero fiber with artificially created liquid oils and semi-hydrogenated oils, which negatively affect the brain and cause damage to the brain. Most packaged foods contain chemicals, preservatives, artificial ingredients, colorants, flavors, textures, and stabilizers.
- *Red Meat and Bacon-* Red meat and bacon are cancer-causing foods or carcinogenic. They are also linked to inflammatory markers. They can be difficult to digest, worsening the leaky gut symptom.
- *Eggs-* Eggs from chickens are genetically modified soy, wheat, and corn. And sometimes are injected with antibiotics.
- *Sucrose and high-fructose corn syrup-* Sucrose can be found in cookies, bread, coffee, cakes, and cereals and is sweetened with brown or white sugar. Food manufacturers add chemically produced sugar to tomato sauce, beverages, and salad dressing.

Excess sugar can cause fatty liver, inflammation, insulin resistance, high cholesterol, and an increase in cancer cells.

How your Gut Flora Can Make You Fat and Brain Sick

Obesity is increasing in numbers all over the world, and this is not something that should be brushed aside. Obesity leads to many health consequences like cancer, diabetes, kidney disease, cardiovascular diseases, osteoarthritic, and neurodegenerative ailments such as Alzheimer's disease. Being overweight increases your chances of depression, cognitive decline, loss of brain tissue, dementia, and other brain diseases. The impact of obesity on the brain should not be underestimated. According to research published in 2014 in the Journal Cell, obesity during pregnancy may cause the fetus to develop abnormal neuronal circuits that control appetite, and this puts the baby at a greater risk of diabetes and weight gain in the later years of the child. Also, the University of Oregon published a paper in 2014 that discovered that obesity during pregnancy could harm the developing fetus stem cells, which create and sustain lifelong blood and immune system function.

Fat Tribes and Thin Tribes

Firmicutes and Bacteroidetes are the two largest groups of bacteria. These two groups make up about ninety percent of the gut's population. The ratio of these groups determines inflammation levels and is related to health conditions like obesity, coronary artery diseases, diabetes, etc. There is no perfect ratio between the two groups, but it is known that the higher the number of firmicutes to bacteroidetes, the higher the risks of inflammation and obesity. Firmicutes are quick to extract calories from food which increases caloric absorption. If your body can absorb more calories from your food as it passes through the gastrointestinal tract, you are at a greater risk of weight gain. However, Bacteroides break down fibers and bulky plant starches into shorter fatty acid molecules that can be utilized by the body for energy.

A study published by Harvard revealed that the Western gut was dominated by firmicutes, and the African gut was dominated by bacteroidetes. One thing about firmicutes is that they regulate human metabolic genes. When these bacteria are abundant in overweight people, they control the genes that adversely impact metabolism. That is, they hijack the DNA and create situations where the body thinks it needs to consume more calories.

Obesity, depression, and dementia are all inflammatory diseases. Obesity is associated with increased production of pro-inflammatory chemicals or cytokines. These molecules are a result of the fat tissue itself, which behaves like an organ pumping out hormones and inflammatory substances. Fat cells not only store extra calories; they are far more involved in human physiology. If you have more fat than you need stored in your visceral organs such as kidneys, liver, heart, intestine, and pancreas, there will be problems with your metabolism. Visceral fats are mostly found in obese individuals, and this can cause a lot of problems. It can activate signaling molecules that meddle with the body's normal hormonal dynamics, and eventually, the visceral fats get inflamed. Additionally, when the visceral fats produce hormonal and inflammatory molecules, they get deposited into the liver, which reacts with another round of ammunition, particularly inflammation-producing reactions, and hormone-disrupting substances. Visceral fats are a dangerous enemy and are linked to several terrible health conditions, such as obesity, cancer, autoimmune disease, and brain disease.

Blood-Sugar and the Brain

Insulin plays a major role in your metabolism by guiding energy from food into cells for their use. The cells in your body can only accept glucose with the help of insulin. Insulin is produced in the pancreas, and it acts as a transporter. It transports glucose from the bloodstream and into the cell to be used as fuel. A healthy and normal cell contains abundant receptors for insulin; it has no problem responding to it. However, when a cell is exposed to the unlimited presence of glucose which is caused by consuming too many carbohydrates and refined sugar, it reacts brilliantly. The cell lowers the amount of insulin-responsive receptors on its surfaces. This situation can be likened to the cell closing a few doors, so it cannot hear insulin knocking. This eventually causes the cell to be resistant or desensitized to insulin. Once a cell becomes insulin-resistant, it will no longer be able to receive glucose from the blood. Therefore, glucose will be left in the bloodstream.

A 'fail-safe' backup system exists whereby the body wants to fix the problem because glucose cannot linger in the blood for too long. So, the body tells the pancreas to produce more insulin to get rid of the glucose. The pancreas continues to pump out higher levels of insulin to push the glucose into the cells because the cells are not as responsive to insulin as before. This process leads to type 2 diabetes.

Type 2 diabetes occurs when you consume immoderate amounts of refined carbohydrates found in bagels, cakes, bread, parathas, and theplas. Consumption of this causes an imbalance of your digestive microbes, which causes cravings, and this leads to a domino effect, which causes blood sugar levels to increase in your bloodstream. When this happens, the pancreas is compelled to work harder to release more insulin to control and manage the sudden rise in the blood sugar level. A diabetic person is someone who has a high blood sugar level because their body cannot ferry glucose into the cells. And the longer the glucose stays in the blood, the more damage it will cause to the body. Diabetes can lead to kidney disease, stroke, blindness, and Alzheimer's disease. Although most people who have diabetes are overweight, many non-overweight people also have diabetes.

Insulin plays a role in the body's reaction when blood sugar levels cannot be managed well. As a so-called anabolic hormone, it promotes fat formation and retention, encourages cellular growth, and stimulates further inflammation. If you have high levels of hormones in your body, it will turn down other hormones, thereby throwing off the body's hormonal system balance. This imbalance has several adverse effects on the body.

An upsurge in blood sugar causes the depletion of important neurotransmitters like serotonin, epinephrine, norepinephrine, GABA, and dopamine. It also causes magnesium levels to sink, which impairs both the nervous system and liver and sparks a reaction called glycation, a biological process where sugar molecules bind proteins and certain fats to form lethal new structures called AGEs which contribute to the degeneration of the brain, and its functioning. It can also cause shrinkage of the brain's critical tissues. Also, insulin resistance can culminate in the formation of those infamous plaques that can be found in Alzheimer's brains. Therefore, obese people are at a greater risk of developing impaired brain function and Alzheimer's disease.

Diabetes and Alzheimer's disease occur due to dietary attacks on the body, which force the body to adjust by developing biological pathways that eventually cause dysfunction and, later on, illness. Diabetes and blood sugar issues below the threshold for diabetes are associated with accelerated risks for brain shrinkage and Alzheimer's disease. There is a relationship between high carbohydrate consumption and diabetes. So, the body underuses insulin that floats around with blood glucose build-up in the bloodstream. They include simple carbohydrates like desserts, baked snacks, and sugary beverages. This leads to the glucose not being able to be broken down, and this starves your body of energy. For example, you may gain weight and have enough stored fats, but you might still feel lethargic. This often means the pancreas has been overworked and may eventually stop working.

How to Avoid Type 2 Diabetes

- Avoid eating refined carbohydrates and stick to fibers. Consume more cruciferous greens, complex grains, seeds, nuts, and fibrous fruits.
- Stay away from junk food. You can do this by not buying them and keeping them around the house, office, or car.
- Have a fixed eating routine and portion and stick to it.
- Spend thirty to forty minutes on aerobics or cardio exercise daily to control blood sugar levels.
- Eat root vegetables and tubers like carrots, artichokes, sweet potatoes, turnips, and parsnips.
- Take pre-biotic supplements to boost your microbes which will help your digestive system.

Chapter Seven

———— · · ● · · ————

The First Brain and

Cognition

The simple definition of cognition is thinking. Cognition refers to the mental skills required to understand the world and carry out simple and complex tasks. According to the National Institute of Aging, cognition can be defined as the capacity to think, learn, and remember. It forms the basis for how we reason, concentrate, plan, organize, and judge. As we get older, we must maintain good cognitive health to continue to stay active and independent. Some declines in cognition and memory with age are normal. However, sometimes, they might signify problems.

Cognitive abilities or brain functions include:

- **Perception-** Refers to how our senses recognize and assimilate information.

- **Attention-** This is the capacity to remain focused on something while filtering out competing thoughts or sensory simulation in the environment. Also, it involves reduction skills.

- **Memory-** Memory could be short or long-term. Short-term memory can be as long as twenty seconds. For example, short-term memory can be used in reading a step-by-step recipe. On the other hand, long-term memory stores information for many years.

- **Motor Skills-** Motor skills are not always considered cognitive abilities. However, it uses brain power, and loss of motor skills can be a part of the effects of cognitive decline. Motor skills aid in the movement of muscles and manipulating objects at will.

- **Language Skills-** Language skills aid in translating sounds into words and generating verbal responses.

- **Visuospatial Processing-** Visuospatial processing is the ability to see objects and understand the spatial relationship that exists between them. For example, the ability to tell how far apart two objects are when placed near each other and whether they are lying at the same or different angles.

- **Executive Functioning-** Executive functioning involves the ability to reason, plan, and take action.

Cognitive Decline

At some point in life, cognition begins to decline with age. Age-related cognitive decline is considered normal. Mild cognitive impairment (MCI) and neurodegenerative conditions like Alzheimer's disease and dementia are not considered normal changes. Normal changes could include a steady deterioration in conceptual reasoning, memory (not remembering recently learned information), and processing speed (slow response to green light).

The 2013 neuroscience research of the Clinics in General Medicine showed that the brain's normal aging might show some signs of cognitive wear and tear caused by the changes to white matter and loss of gray matter volume. The brain contains about 60% white matter and 40% gray matter. All the processing goes on in the gray matter, while the white matter allows communication between all the different gray areas and the other parts of the body. Gray matter can be seen as a factory, and white matter can be seen as a truck that transports goods from one factory to another.

Gray matter starts to decline after age twenty, particularly at the prefrontal cortex and hippocampus. Scientists believe that this decline may be a result of dying neurons. Amyloid Beta is a component of the amyloid plaques found in the brains of people suffering from a protein found in all people suffering from Alzheimer's disease. Also, it can be that it is because neurons grow smaller, and the connections between them decline. As one age, neurons become smaller, simpler, and shorter and become less connected to one another. Aging brings about shrinkage in white and gray matter, and white matter shrinks much more than gray matter.

Age-related cognitive decline is not as serious as MCI. Age-related cognitive decline affects thinking and memory. The decline happens so that it is enough to be noticed but not to the extent that it interferes with daily life. Some causes of cognitive impairment (such as depression, medication side effects, and vitamin B12 deficiency) are treatable. Cognitive impairment does not always lead to Alzheimer's disease, unlike MCI, which is a major risk factor for Alzheimer's disease.

Dementia

Dementia is a global issue and is gradually becoming more common among people, and it is present in many families or among people they know. Dementia is not a single disease but a clinical syndrome that is a collection of symptoms and other attributes that co-exist and develop a recognized pattern. That is, dementia is a term used to describe the symptoms of brain disorders like stroke, Alzheimer's disease, etc. Some dementia symptoms include problems with memory, language, thinking, and social behavior changes. Dementia is not caused by aging, even though it is more common in older adults. Problem recalling a word, irregular forgetfulness, or other symptoms might just be a normal part of aging and may not be linked to dementia.

Alzheimer Disease

The most common form of dementia is Alzheimer's disease, and it is responsible for about 60%-80% of all cases of dementia, either on its own or with other forms of pathology. The disease was named after a German psychiatrist, Alois Alzheimer when he described the disease over one hundred years ago. Alzheimer's disease is a permanent, progressive brain disorder that is the sixth leading cause of death in the United States.

In the early stages of the disease, the patient has difficulty finding words and remembering recent events. As the disease advances, greater memory loss and language difficulties will become more apparent. The early symptoms for most people with Alzheimer's disease appear much later in life, after age sixty-five. According to the National Institute of Aging, Alzheimer's might result from a combination of factors such as the environment, genetics, and lifestyle. Alzheimer's disease mostly occurs in people between the ages of thirty to sixty. It is predominantly related to a family history of early onset. Although, sometimes, it appears without any known cause. There is an abnormal deposition of amyloid plaques, neurofibrillary tangles, synaptic loss, neuronal loss, inflammation, and brain atrophy in the brain. These abnormal plaques and tangles interrupt and meddle with the normal functioning of the brain cells. The accumulation of amyloid-β peptide is the primary component of amyloid plaques which is presumed to lead to a pathogenic cascade that ultimately leads to Alzheimer's disease.

The APOE gene provides the instructions required to make the apolipoprotein E protein. This protein combines with fats or lipids in the body to develop molecules called lipoproteins. Lipoproteins package the cholesterol and other fats in the body and carry them through the bloodstream. Maintaining normal cholesterol levels is important to prevent disorders affecting the heart and blood vessels. The APOE gene has three slightly different types (alleles) called e2, e3, and e4. The most common allele is e3 and is predominantly found in more than half of the general population.

The e4 allele increases a person's risk for developing late-onset Alzheimer's disease. Individuals who inherit one copy of the e4 allele have a higher chance of developing the disease, and those who inherit two copies are at even higher risk. The e4 allele may be associated with the earlier onset of memory loss and other symptoms compared to people with Alzheimer's disease who do not have this allele.

Apolipoprotein E genotyping is a laboratory test that helps to ascertain the diagnosis of late-onset Alzheimer's disease in adults who display the symptoms. However, it cannot be used alone. And there are no definite tests for Alzheimer's disease. The test is only appropriate for screening those who show symptoms and not appropriate for those without symptoms. All cases of Alzheimer's disease are due to cognitive decline, but not all cognitive decline is due to Alzheimer's disease.

Some Risk Factors for Late-onset Alzheimer's Disease

- Genetic factors (especially with the presence of the e4 allele of the APOE gene)
- Family history
- Aging
- Midlife hypertension
- Obesity
- History of head trauma
- Diabetes
- Hypercholesterolemia

Some researchers believe that eating unhealthy foods, pollution, illness, and smoking causes oxidative stress and inflammation, which is the primary cause of Alzheimer's disease. A healthy person's blood-brain barrier protects the brain from oxidative stress and inflammation. However, the blood-brain barrier deteriorates in the early stages of Alzheimer's disease.

Vascular Dementia

Vascular dementia occurs when the blood supply to the brain is jeopardized by an arterial disease that reduces neuronal function and causes the death of brain cells. Vascular dementia can occur after a stroke blocks an artery in the brain. Although strokes do not always cause vascular dementia, it can be due to other conditions that destroy blood vessels and decrease circulation, which prevents vital oxygen and nutrients from reaching the brain.

Dementia with Lewy Bodies

This is the third most common type of dementia, accounting for about ten percent of dementia cases. It is linked to Parkinson's and Alzheimer's diseases because they have similar characteristics. Lewy bodies are small accumulations of alpha-synuclein protein, which occur in the cells in several brain parts. As seen in Alzheimer's disease, it can lead to memory loss. Also, it could lead to planning difficulty, disorientation to space, and difficulty in establishing alertness. As seen in Parkinson's disease, Lewy bodies can lead to trembling limbs and reduced facial expressions. Dementia with Lewy Bodies causes recurrent falls, hallucinations, nightmares/disturbed sleep, and fluctuations in levels of conscious awareness.

Frontotemporal Dementia

This is a fairly uncommon type of dementia, affecting regions in the brain's frontal part responsible for language, planning, motivation, and emotions. There are many types of frontotemporal dementia, and they depend on the part of the frontal or temporal lobe affected. It may lead to behavioral changes (behavioral variant frontotemporal dementia) and language and speech (primary progressive aphasia). Behavioral changes might affect the patient's personality. They might lead to a lack of empathy, inhibitions, difficulty in planning, preference for sweet foods, overeating, and adoption of rigid routines due to the lack of mental flexibility. Language problems may lead to semantic dementia and difficulty in producing speech.

Mixed Dementia

This is a condition that involves more than one type of dementia. For example, a case of mixed Alzheimer's and vascular dementia involves clinical features and changes in the brain peculiar to both conditions. Mixed dementia occurs mostly with aging beyond eighty years. Therefore, a mixture of Alzheimer's and vascular pathology is mostly discovered during the autopsy. It is mostly characterized by a slow decline in abilities and strokes.

Some less Common Causes of Dementia

Huntington's Disease- This disease is an autosomal dominant inherited disease that leads to an anomaly in movement and coordination difficulties as well as cognitive problems. It usually starts in middle age. Cognitive problems appear in the early stages, while dementia occurs later on in people with advanced Huntington's disease.

Multiple Sclerosis- This occurs when multiple sclerosis affects specific areas of the brain leading to cognitive difficulties among people over a period. Particularly, the extent of frontal lobe atrophy may predict the extent of cognitive impairment.

Corticobasal Degeneration- This damages and shrinks the brain due to abnormal protein deposits in the brain. This leads to loss of balance and dementia.

Human Immunodeficiency Virus (HIV) related Dementia- Dementia can occur due to the direct infection of the brain due to HIV or lack of immunity, which leads to cancers and other brain infections. Neurocognitive disorders are still very common in people with HIV despite the advancement of antiretroviral therapies.

Creutzfeldt-Jakob disease- This disease is caused by infectious protein particles found inside the brain. These protein particles are referred to as prions. Creutzfeldt–Jakob disease affects one in a million people, and it takes many years before an infected person starts exhibiting symptoms. Firstly, symptoms start with lethargy, memory lapses, and mood disturbances. The disease advances to loss of balance and eventually death. Death is likely to occur within six months of exhibiting early symptoms.

Normal Pressure Hydrocephalus- This disease occurs when excess fluid accumulates in the brain cavities, which exerts pressure on the brain. Some of the symptoms include urinary incontinence, loss of balance, and cognitive problems. Although there is a paucity of controlled trials, it seems that this disease can be improved by neurosurgery. However, it seems dementia appears to be least likely to improve.

Risk Factors for Dementia

Age- Age is a significant and constant risk factor for dementia. The number of new occurrences at a given time and the number of cases at any time double every five years at the age of sixty-five to eighty-five. This does not necessarily mean that dementia is mainly caused by age and that everyone in that age bracket is prone to have dementia. However, age is just a bigger risk factor to consider when dealing with dementia.

Genes- Although several genes are known to be linked to Alzheimer's disease, not all cause Alzheimer's disease, so much to lead to an increase in susceptibility; if you have a first-degree relative with late-onset Alzheimer's disease, your chances of having Alzheimer's disease increase.

Gender- More men develop vascular dementia than women. Also, Alzheimer's disease is more common in women than men.

Down's syndrome- Three copies of chromosome 21 are usually found in people suffering from Down's syndrome. Down's syndrome carries the genes that are linked with amyloid production, which may be the reason most but not all people with Down's syndrome develop Alzheimer's disease in middle age.

Depression- A complex relationship exists between dementia and depression. Studies have found that depression is usually one of the first symptoms of dementia long before memory changes are noticed. Depression is established in most dementia cases because of the losses in the patient's experiences and brain changes. Depressed people find it difficult to remember things and depressed people have higher risks of dementia.

Vascular Dementia Risk Factors

Stroke- This is a vital risk factor in vascular dementia, and researchers opine that it also increases the risks of Alzheimer's disease.

Blood Pressure- High blood pressure is a risk factor for stroke and can cause vascular dementia. It can also lead to Alzheimer's disease.

Diabetes Mellitus- Diabetes mellitus increases a patient's chance of having dementia due to the harmful impact of high blood glucose on the brain and the effect of diabetes on small blood vessels. It can also lead to heart disease and hypertension.

Heart Disease- Heart conditions like irregular heart rhythm and heart failure are linked to an increased risk of dementia.

Smoking- Your lifestyle can also influence the probability of developing dementia. It also negatively affects the blood vessels in the brain, leading to higher risks of vascular dementia.

Chapter Eight

· —— · · ● · · —— ·

The MIND Diet

MIND is an abbreviation for 'Mediterranean-DASH Intervention for Neurodegenerative Delay.' DASH is an acronym for 'Dietary Approaches to Stop Hypertension.' The MIND diet combines the Mediterranean and DASH to create a dietary plan that centers specifically on the brain. It is a healthy eating way designed to help fight Alzheimer's disease and other cognitive problems. Studies have revealed that this diet keeps the brain seven and a half years younger and lowers the vulnerability of developing Alzheimer's disease and other cognitive problems by fifty-three percent. It also reduces blood pressure risks of heart disease, diabetes, and many other diseases. Many studies have shown that combining foods from Mediterranean and DASH diets has various positive benefits on brain development and health.

The MIND diet was created by Harvard University and Rush University Medical Center (RUMC) researchers. The research team was led by Dr. Martha Clare Morris, the director of nutritional epidemiology in the Department of Internal Medicine at RUMC in Chicago. The diet was designed to improve brain health. The diet is built on the basis that foods needed to enrich the brain are taken from the two well-established diets supported by nutrition and dementia research.

The MIND diet consists of fifteen components. These components include the ten best MIND diets to consume for a healthy brain and the five worst diets to avoid.

Brain Healthy Foods

The healthy brain food groups include;

Green and Leafy Vegetables- green leafy vegetables provide folate, vitamin E, carotenoids, and flavonoids. Eat about six or more servings per week. Examples include spinach, salads, kale, and cooked greens.

All other vegetables- avoid starchy vegetables because the non-starchy ones provide several nutrients for a low level of calories. Non-starchy vegetables are higher in fiber and lower in sugar than starchy vegetables. Examples of starchy vegetables include corn, green peas, and sweet and white potatoes. Examples of non-starchy vegetables include eggplant and black olives.

Nuts- eat about five or more servings per week. Healthy nuts include almonds, pine nuts, hazelnuts, pistachios, Brazil nuts, walnuts, pecans, and cashew nuts.

Berries- eat berries at least twice each week. Examples include; strawberries, raspberries, blackberries, and blueberries. These berries all have antioxidant benefits.

Olive oil- Olive oil should be used mainly for cooking. Olive oil is extremely healthy because it contains powerful antioxidants and beneficial fatty acids. However, many believe the oil is unsuitable for cooking because of its unsaturated fat content. Others believe it is good for cooking and frying. Extra virgin oil is the best olive oil to use.

Fish- Fish should be eaten at least once per week. Fatty fishes like sardines, trout, salmon, mackerel, and tuna are best because of their high amounts of omega-3 fatty acids. It is common knowledge that frying is not the healthiest way of preparing a meal. Frying increases saturated fat intake and reduces omega-3 fat levels. Avoid or limit eating fried fish and opt for baked, cooked, or steamed fish instead.

Whole grains- eat three servings daily. Examples of whole grains include quinoa, brown rice, oatmeal, whole-grain pasta, and whole-grain bread.

Beans- beans should be eaten at least four times per week. They include; lentils, soybeans, and beans.

Poultry- chicken or turkey should be eaten at least twice per week. Fried chicken or turkey is not encouraged on the MIND diet.

Wine- one glass of wine per day. Red and white wine are good for the brain.

Do not quit the MIND diet if consuming the target servings is difficult. Studies have shown that if the MIND diet is followed to a certain extent, then it can still reduce the risk of Alzheimer's disease and cognitive impairment.

Brain Harming Foods

The MIND diet brain-harming foods include butter and margarine, whole-fat cheese, red meat, fried fast food, and pastries and sweets. Limiting or avoiding these foods was part of the MIND studies, and it was found that there was better cognitive aging and a reduced vulnerability to Alzheimer's disease. These foods lead to blood-brain barrier problems, which lead to an increase in beta-amyloid plaque. Our body produces all the saturated fats that the body needs; there is no biological need to have saturated fats in our diet. Therefore, consuming unsaturated fats instead, like polyunsaturated type, reduces LDL cholesterol and heart attack. Also, consuming monosaturated fats like nuts and olive oils instead of saturated fats provides several benefits.

It is recommended to limit or avoid the following foods during the MIND diet;

Butter and Margarine- the MIND diet suggests eating less than one tablespoon daily. This diet suggests using olive oil as the main fat and for cooking. Generally, fats at solid temperatures have too much saturated fat to be included in the MIND diet—foods like coconut oil, palm oil, beef tallow, lard, and shortening. Vegetable oil spreads with zero Trans fats and lower saturated fat should be used instead of butter and margarine.

Cheese- the MIND diet recommends eating less than one portion (1½ oz) of cheese each week. The dietary guidelines for Americans and the American Heart Association recommend limiting cheese for a healthy heart diet. The MIND diet suggests eating low-fat or fat-free milk or yogurt instead of whole-fat cheese to lower sodium and saturated fat intake while benefitting from potassium, vitamins A, and D in dairy foods. You can also opt for vegan cheese because it offers zero cholesterol. However, they may still be high in saturated fats.

Red Meat- red meat includes lamb, beef, pork, and duck. They can be found in foods like burritos, sausages, meatballs, meatloaf, hamburgers, beef tacos, and hot dogs. The MIND diet recommends not eating red meat no more than four times each week. The World

Health Organization has classified processed meat as a group 1 carcinogen which is in the same category as tobacco and asbestos. If you have not started eating red meat, then there is no reason for you to start incorporating it into your diet. And if you love red meat and cannot stop eating it, the following are ways in which you can eat red meat in the healthiest possible ways;

- Select the leased processed meat. Pick fresh-cut meats, unlike processed meats like bacon, bologna, hot dogs, beef jerky, ham, pepperoni, and sausages.
- Go for grass-fed, organic meat because they are leaner and include more vitamin E, zinc, iron, potassium, and carotenoids.
- Select meat with the lowest percentage of fats in regards to ground meat.

Fried Food- the MIND diet recommends limiting eating fried foods, especially the ones from fast-food restaurants, to no more than once weekly. This is because frying diminishes the healthiness of any food. It dilutes the nutrients in already healthy foods like poultry, vegetables, and fish, negatively affecting brain health.

Pastries and Sweets- the MIND diet recommends eating no more than five times weekly. These foods not only contain bad fat but also added sugar. There is no need for these foods to be added to your diet because they offer no positive nutrients. And if you must eat them, they should be eaten in limited amounts. They include processed snacks and desserts, and they include ice cream, doughnuts, custards, croissants, candy, cakes, and brownies. Also, sugar-sweetened beverages, like sports drinks, soda, and juice which are not one hundred percent juice, should be limited. Whole fruits naturally contain sugar in a reasonable, and they can be used to satisfy your sweet tooth.

These brain-harming foods above contain saturated fats and Trans fats which are known to cause several diseases like Alzheimer's disease. To earn a diet score of fifteen in the MIND diet, you should eat at least three servings of whole grains, one serving of vegetables, and one glass of wine daily. It also means that you will eat leafy greens almost every day, nuts at least five times per week, beans four times a week, berries twice per week, poultry twice a week, fish once a week, and olive oil as the major cooking oil. Also, you will have to limit the foods that are not good for brain development and health. That is, you will eat less than one tablespoon of butter or margarine per day, consume pastries and sweets less than five times a week, red meat not more than four times a week, less than one serving of whole-fat cheese per week, and less than one fast fried food per week. Each of these requirements earns you one point, which equals fifteen points.

The MIND diet is not as demanding as the Mediterranean or DASH diet because it requires fewer servings of fish, fruits, vegetables, and grains with no emphasis on limiting dairy or total fats. The diet is different because it recommends green and leafy vegetables. However, it does not recommend fruits other than berries, like blackberries, strawberries, pomegranates, blueberries, and raspberries.

The MIND diet uses an evidence-based approach to select anti-inflammatory and antioxidant foods that protect the brain and make it difficult for plaques to be formed. Limiting brain-damaging foods is very important because they damage the blood-brain barrier and promote the formation of damaging beta-amyloid plaques.

Before the MIND diet came into play, the Mediterranean and DASH diets were studied in other to understand how the diets can benefit human health. The Mediterranean diet is plant-based and focuses on vegetables, fruits, beans, whole grains, legumes, olive oil, herbs and spices, and seafood. In moderation, it recommends poultry, eggs, yogurt, cheese, and optional wine. And it limits sweets and red meat. Several studies have found this diet to be beneficial to heart health and diabetes. As I already mentioned above, you can find more information about the Mediterranean Diet in a book written by Emma Collins, INTERMITTENT   FASTING   FOR   WOMEN   AND

MEDITERRANEAN DIET FOR BEGINNERS: The Complete Guide on How to Lose Weight and Increase Longevity.

The DASH diet is also plant-based and designed to decrease blood pressure. It focuses on fruits, vegetables, seeds, legumes, grains, and low-fat, with occasional poultry, lean meat, and fish. Studies have revealed that the DASH diet reduces blood pressure, lowers harmful LDL cholesterol and triglycerides, and increases beneficial HDL cholesterol.

The Mediterranean and the DASH diet are not the same. The Mediterranean diet focuses on olive oil as the major fat, is high in fish, and includes a moderate amount of wine with foods. The DASH diet is different from the Mediterranean diet because the diet does not particularly recommend dairy, fruit, or multiple fish a week, but it specifically recommends green, leafy vegetables and berries.

Studies have shown that the risks of Alzheimer's disease can be cut by thirty-five to fifty-three percent when following the MIND diet. In 2015, a study was taken to determine the link between cognitive decline and the MIND diet. Nine hundred and twenty-three people between the ages of fifty-eight and ninety-eight took part in the RUMC Memory and Aging Project (MAP). MAP compared how well their diets matched the DASH, Mediterranean, and MIND diets and how much was linked to Alzheimer's disease. The sample population lived in Chicago's senior public housing units or retirement areas. These people were tested at least twice to be certain that they did not have Alzheimer's disease before the commencement of the study. One hundred and forty-four new cases of Alzheimer's disease were discovered throughout four and a half years of follow-up.

A wide range of results was discovered regarding how the participants' diets resonated with the Mediterranean, DASH, and MIND diets. This helped discover how a group of foods was associated with Alzheimer's disease. The results were divided into three categories, and the top scores were linked to healthy meals.

The first group was the MIND diet, and the participants' diets were based on a total possible score of fifteen. One point was given to each of the fifteen MIND diet components. The top third of scores averaged 9.6 on the 15-point MIND scale, and the results ranged from 8.5 to 12.5. The middle third of the scores averaged 7.5, ranging from 7 to 8 points. These groups had a considerably lesser risk of developing Alzheimer's disease. Risks were cut by 53 and 35% for the top third and middle third, respectively. For the Mediterranean diet, the top third of scores cut risks by fifty-four percent, while the top third for the DASH diet was associated with a significant risk reduction, though it was lower than thirty-nine percent. It was observed that strictly following the DASH diet was not as protective as the other diets. What was unique to the DASH diet was dairy and low salt, and researchers agreed that the guidelines were not specifically important for brain health. This means that following the Mediterranean or DASH diet has benefits, but the MIND diet has great benefits even when followed halfway. Additionally, the MIND diet is less demanding and stressful in many ways. It requires fewer servings of grains, fish, vegetables, and fruits, and there is no focus on dairy or limitations on total fats.

The researchers found that the MIND diet was fairly protective in the participants with a probable genetic marker for late-onset Alzheimer's disease.

MIND Diet and Nutrients

Understanding the key functions of nutrients will improve your understanding of food and how you can improve your brain and overall body health. This section is all about the knowledge about the best nutrients that are involved in cognitive aging, cognitive development, and dementia, as well as anti-inflammatory nutrients and antioxidants that protect the brain against beta-amyloid deposits and cell death.

Good and Bad Fat

The PREDIMED trial tested the Mediterranean diet with healthy fats like olive oil and nuts, and both were very effective in improving cognitive scores compared to low-fat diets. This shows a lower risk of Alzheimer's disease and cognitive decline when unsaturated fats are used instead of saturated or trans fats. The MIND diet emphasizes the use of olive oils as the major dietary fat because it is rich in monounsaturated fat and polyphenols. Healthy fats can also be obtained from vegetable oil, seeds, nuts, and avocado.

Bad Fats

Consuming excess trans and saturated fats accelerates the risks of dementia. Diets rich in these fats cause blood-brain barrier dysfunction, amyloid clusters, and inflammation. The easiest way to avoid saturated and trans fats is to stick to the MIND diet and avoid brain-harming foods. A good way to identify saturated fat is to observe and check if it becomes solid at room temperature.

Vitamin E

MIND diet that naturally contains vitamin E includes olive oil, green and leafy vegetables, nuts, and whole grains. Vitamin E is an antioxidant nutrient vital to brain health because it defends the brain from oxidative stress and damage to neural tissue resulting from high metabolic activity. Deficiency in vitamin E brings about several brain-related problems like cognitive decline, decreased sensitivity to vibration, lack of reflexes, loss of control over body movement, and paralyzed eye muscles.

Vitamin E is a collective term for a family of eight naturally occurring homologs with powerful antioxidant properties. They occur in two groups; four tocopherols and four tocotrienols, each of which has an alpha, beta, gamma, and delta. They include alpha-, beta-, gamma-, and delta-tocopherol and alpha-, beta-, gamma-, and delta-tocotrienol, and they all have varying levels of biological activities. For this book, only two will be studied. And they include alpha-tocopherol and gamma-tocopherol. Both forms of vitamin E can be found in foods with antioxidant and inflammatory properties. However, most of the vitamin E on food labels is alpha-tocopherol because it is the most common form in food supplements.

Vitamin E has been proposed as a possible clinical intervention for Alzheimer's disease because of the reliability of its several biological functions, which affect the neurodegenerative processes associated with Alzheimer's disease. Vitamin E has a wide range of biological functions, and they differ according to their form. Tocopherol and tocotrienol have several properties and functions associated with the chemical saturation level in their molecular structures, with tocopherols having phytyl side chains and tocotrienols having three carbon-carbon double bonds.

Vitamin E from foods is better than the ones gotten from supplements because they gotten from a supplement may do more harm than good. This is because the amounts of vitamin E in foods are moderate and work as a team to keep the brain healthy. Also, the foods consumed may contain all the forms of vitamin E.

Vitamin E is an essential element that the body cannot produce; it must come from your diet. Its antioxidant properties mean that it protects your body from the harm caused by free radicals, keeps the immune strong and healthy helps the body use vitamin K, helps form red blood cells, and helps widen the blood vessels to prevent blood from clotting inside them. Also, it is fat-soluble, meaning the body needs dietary fat to absorb it.

For your eating pattern to be healthy, your diet must include at least twenty percent of calories from fats. If not, it won't be easy to meet the recommended intake levels of vital fat-soluble nutrients. The type of fat consumed in the body is more important than the total fat consumed as long as a particular minimum (20%) is met and is within calorie needs.

B Vitamins; Folate (B9) and (Cobalamin) B12

Vitamin B9 and B12 are both essential, water-soluble B vitamins, which means that it is not usually stored in the body, and the excesses are removed in the urine. They are usually discussed together because they are interrelated and perform many of the same functions. The body's red blood cell count goes down if either is absent, which reduces the ability to send oxygen to the tissues in the body. Vitamin B12 deficiency can cause cognitive impairment, depression, fatigue, anemia, and nerve damage leading to tingling, burning, numbness, and peripheral neuropathy. Vitamin B9 and B12 are involved in brain development in the early stages of one's life and brain degeneration in later life. These two vitamins are vital for the brain because they help metabolize homocysteine, a substance linked to Alzheimer's disease. Without vitamins B9 and B12, homocysteine begins to accumulate in the body. A study by the National Health and Nutrition Examination Survey (NHANES) found that low levels of B12 and folate led to impaired cognitive performance compared to people with normal folate levels.

Vitamin B12 is not well absorbed by thirty percent of older adults because their stomach becomes less acidic with aging. Still, because B12 can be stored in the liver for up to three to five years, cognitive decline and damage could develop years before the signs of anemia appear. Folate deficiency or B12 speeds up cognitive decline, and low folate may lead to Alzheimer's disease. Consuming excess folate can speed up cognitive decline, especially if you have low levels of B12. Folate naturally obtained from foods would not lead to an increase in high levels, but folate obtained from supplements and foods produced with fortified grains will lead to high folate intake. People already getting enough folate and B12 from food will not necessarily benefit more from adding vitamins as a supplement. Foods containing folate include dark green vegetables like spinach, artichokes, collard greens, broccoli, and Brussels sprouts, and legumes like chickpeas, beans, peas, and edamame. Vitamin B12 is found in animal foods like fish and poultry. It is also found in some fortified milk alternatives (almond milk, soy milk, and rice milk) and soy-based meat alternatives.

Flavonoids and Carotenoids

The brain is constantly busy, and all metabolic activities put the brain at risk of oxidative stress and tissue damage. Antioxidant enzymes in the body are not always available to the brain, like antioxidant nutrients from food, which makes them more important to the aging brain. Flavonoids and carotenoids are other classes of antioxidants that can help the brain. The MIND diet recommends plenty of flavonoids and carotenoids, which can be found in berries and leafy greens.

Flavonoids are biologically active polyphenolic compounds crucial for good health, and they occur naturally in a wide range of plant foods like vegetables, fruits, nuts, tea, and wine. There are six main subclasses of flavonoids: anthocyanidins, flavan-3-ols, flavonols, flavones, flavanones, and isoflavones. Major sources of flavonoids include:

- Berries like strawberries, elderberries, blueberries, raspberries, and European black currants.
- Vegetables like purple cabbage and eggplants.
- Whole grains like quinoa.
- Beans like garbanzo beans.
- Other foods like oranges, onion, grapefruit, black tea, green tea, oolong tea, tomatoes, bananas, lemons, and parsley.

Carotenoids are naturally occurring orange, yellow/green, and red pigments made by plants, most of which have antioxidant properties. Examples of carotenoids include alpha-carotene, beta-carotene, lycopene, lutein, Zeaxanthin, and beta-cryptoxanthin. Consuming carotenoid foods has been linked to a reduced risk of cardiovascular disease, some cancers, cataracts, and age-related macular degeneration. They are best absorbed with fats like olive oil.

Some sources of carotenoids include leafy greens like collard greens, spinach, and kale; vegetables like carrots, red bell pepper, pumpkin, and sweet potato; nuts like pistachios; Brussels sprouts and broccoli; and other fruits like watermelon, cantaloupe, and apricots.

Chapter Nine

It All Comes Down

to Food

So far, everything that has been discussed in this book points to something, and that is food. Food is the fuel that powers good health. Without food in the body, the body becomes weak until it eventually shuts down. If there is anything that I have done to change my life, it is to take cognizance of the type of food I put into my mouth. I have come to realize that food comes a long way and, when eaten right, solves more than 50% of our problems. The world is filled with so much junk right now, and one thing you have to understand is that sometimes producers are not concerned about how healthy food is. All they are after is money. But you are the only one responsible for your health and not those producers and sellers out there. Work on yourself and always be ready to say no to unhealthy food. It will not be easy at first, but that is where this book comes in. This book is here to show you how to manage your diet to manage your life.

If you are reading this chapter, then you should already know how food impacts your health and what health truly means. Now, you should know that not all foods are good and that understanding the nutritional components of food will go a long way in maintaining good health. Knowledge is power, and consuming as much knowledge about food as possible is advisable. It is never too late to learn. All you have to do is pick up this book and any other book and read to learn. I mentioned a few in this book that you may be interested in. And knowledge will be a complete waste of time if you do not put into practice what you have learned. Practice and consistency work hand in hand. You have to be consistent if you want to see changes. You should draft a plan and work on the plan. Do not start eating vegetables today and then go back to sodas and junk food tomorrow.

Remember to relax! Stress has a way of undoing all your hard work. I recommend taking at least thirty minutes each day to rest. Do not be in a hurry to wake up from bed. Go to bed early enough so that you can wake up the following day without feeling stressed. Take your time to eat! Rushing to have breakfast is very dangerous to your health!

I am very grateful that I have been able to write the last chapter of this book. I can only imagine the health problems several people face daily. I used to be one of those people, and now I know better; it is time to let others know what I have learned over the years. I want this book to be a game changer for your life, as the knowledge poured down into this book was a game changer for me. Now you know that certain brain diseases can be prevented if we incorporate brain-healthy foods. Brain-healthy foods do not only apply to adults but also children believe eating a healthy diet from a young age greatly benefits people as they age.

I hope you had fun reading this book just as much as I had fun writing it?!

BOOK 2

Your 28-Day Meal

Plan

N ow that you have decided to start your 28-day Mind diet meal plan, you must get it right on your first attempt. This book aims to help you eat healthily for the next 28 days. Meal planning is all about selecting the meals you will eat over a period. What this means is that you plan what you will eat for breakfast, lunch, and dinner over a few days, weeks, or months for yourself and your family.

This book has planned your breakfast, lunch, and dinner over 28 days to make your healthy food journey easier. Following this meal plan will save you a lot of time and reduce the time it will take you to shop and think about what to eat. Also, having a meal plan saves money because you get to do your shopping in bulk which saves costs. It also reduces stress because you do not have to decide on a meal to eat when you have organized everything in advance.

Pros of Meal Planning

- Meal planning saves energy, time, and money. Because your meals are already prepared, you do not have to stand in front of the fridge or pantry pondering what to eat. Also, meal planning saves money because you will not have to spend money at restaurants. Meal planning involves purchasing food items in bulk which helps to save money. And sticking to what you have on the list will help you to avoid impulse purchases at the store.

- It allows you to fulfill the nutritional requirements of everyone living in the house.

- It makes food economical.

- Meal Planning Prevents Wastage. This means that you only get to buy the amount of food that you need

- Learn Portion Control. Meal planning will make you know how much food you are consuming, and this prevents you from overeating or undereating.

- Eat Healthily. Meal planning helps you to eat healthily. This is because when you are hungry, your blood sugar drops, and you tend to eat whatever you can get fast. However, with meal planning, you get a balanced meal at your fingertips.

Factors to Consider When Planning Your Meals

When want to create your meal plan, there are several guidelines you need to keep in mind in other to have a successful and effective meal plan.

1. *Time, energy, and skill*

    A very important factor to consider when you are about to create your meal plan is your time, energy, and skill. Do not add elaborate meals you do not have the time or energy to prepare or do not know how to prepare.

2. *Age Factor*

    Your age determines your diet to a large extent, and you must have observed that the diet of various members of different age groups differs. What a small child eats is quite different from what a baby eats, or what an adult eats. Put age into consideration when creating your meal plan.

3. *Nutritional Adequacy*

The nutritional adequacy of everyone in the house should be considered when creating your meal plan. For example, a pregnant woman needs calcium and a growing child needs more protein. Your meal plan should contain food items from various food groups.

4. *Economic Consideration*

When creating your meal plan, ensure that you plan a balanced diet within your budget. You can buy food in bulk and store it in a fridge, purchase from fair-price shops, and don't throw away leftover food.

5. *Availability*

Not all foods are available all year, so you might have to make some changes to your meal plan at some point in the year. Also, off-season foods are usually more expensive and less fresh and nutritious than season foods.

6. *Likes and Dislikes*

It will be difficult to stick to your meal plan if you include most foods that are disliked by members of the family. So, only include liked foods in the meal plan.

Food Safety Rules

- Do not forget to wash your hands thoroughly before you start any food preparation.

- Leftovers should be reheated or refrigerated immediately.

- Defrost frozen foods in a fridge at a temperature that is at or below 5°C. Frozen food should be kept on the bottom shelf so that it does not drip on other foods.

How to Organise a Meal Plan

Meal Ideas

Do not start your meal plan blindly. Write down all the meals you can cook and the ones you cannot cook. There are also resources like this book that will assist you with recipes on your journey. If you do not live alone, collaborate with others living with you so that you can know what they like and what they do not like. This will save you a lot of problems in the long run. When you want to create your meal plan, simply go through your list to make sure that you only incorporate meals that you can prepare.

To help you get started, you can list the meals by category, e.g. poultry. You can also include side dishes and snacks you love and can prepare. This list does not have to be typed and printed, you can just write it down with a pen and jotter. Remember, just keep it simple!

Think Ahead

Check your calendar to know what you are supposed to do each day before creating your meal plan! Decide on the number of days you want to plan. Is it 5 days? 7 days? Look at your schedule and use it to design your meal plan because if you have plans on a particular night, it might prevent you from cooking the food in the meal plan. So, it is best to plan your meal with your schedule. This means that when writing your meal plan, you take into account the time you have available to cook the meal. This is very important because knowing how much time you have available to prepare a meal will help you stick to the meal plan in the long run. On your busy days, opt for easy-to-make dishes that will not cause you a lot of trouble and time to make. For example, you could opt for a simple salad and call it a day! You can also go for leftovers during extra busy days. When you have so much available time, you can prepare complicated and time-consuming meals.

Create the Meal Plan

Now, that you have thought about the available time you have each day, and the meals you can and cannot prepare, it is time to create your meal plan. Look around your kitchen and note the food items you already have and the ones you do not have. Write down all the ingredients you will need to make the recipes and cross off the ones you already have. Make sure you incorporate meals that utilize the ingredients you already have at home to avoid wastage. And if the ingredients are not healthy, feel free to do away with them.

Meal plan time-saving tips

Tips 1: Keep your meal plans in a safe place so that you can reuse them when you want to create another meal plan. Here, you could just make some changes by adding new recipes and taking out some old ones. This tip is very helpful when you do not have the time to create a new meal plan from scratch!

Tip 2: If you do not have the time to create your meal plan, you can also make use of templates online. You just have to search for the ones that suit your family's taste preferences and dietary needs. You can also use meal plan templates to create your own.

Tip 3: Now that it is time to create the meal plan, pick a day or time to create your weekly or monthly meal plan.

Shopping list

Write a concise list so you will not forget to purchase some important ingredients from the store. Your shopping list can be divided into fridge items, cupboard items, freezer items, and others like those below.

FRIDGE	FREEZER	CUPBOARD	OTHERS

Your shopping lists help you to save time, money, and energy and help you to limit distractions. When creating your shopping list, go through your meal plan to know what ingredients are needed in the preparation of the meal. Check if you already have some of the ingredients, and only write the ones you do not have in the list. Some people prefer to use their phones to make their shopping lists, but paper and pen make it easier for you to jot down your lists. Also, decide the best time to go shopping. Make sure you go shopping on the days you have ample amount of time to move around the stores to purchase the items on your lists. Try as much as possible to resist impulse purchases, but if you must buy something on impulse, limit yourself to one or two items, and do not go overboard. When you come back home, ensure that you arrange everything you have bought and put them into the proper place.

How to Save Time While Shopping

- The first step is to clean out your fridge before going to the market. Note the foods you have left and the ones you need. Take out expired and leftover foods you no longer need. Clean out your pantry and check out if you need to throw out some foods you do not need anymore.

- Make a shopping list and do not forget to take it along with you on your way to the market because you might forget what you need and you might purchase things you do not need.

- Fill your stomach before going to the market. Hunger increases your chances of impulse buying and this is not what you want.

- Going to the market alone is the best because it helps you to avoid distraction and temptation and this will help you limit the purchase of unnecessary things.

Prep

To make it easier for you, you can prep your meals during the weekend so that you do not have to spend all day in the kitchen during the week. For example, you can blend your tomatoes, chop your vegetables, and boil or fry your meat and fish. You can also cook over the weekend and freeze your meals to eat during the week.

What You Can Do on Prep Day

- Cut your meat into smaller portions to store in marinades to refrigerate.
- You can also boil or fry the meat before storing it in the refrigerator.
- Chop your fruits and vegetables and store them in the fridge.

- Bake your bread, healthy options of cookies, and any other thing ahead for the week.

- Soak and cook your beans.

- Make your salad dressing.

- Grate your cheese.

- Cook soups and stews.

Don't Forget to Have a Backup Plan

Sometimes, things do not go the way we planned. For example, food may get burnt or spoilt, etc. Always have leftovers from a previous meal on hand just in case you mess up the meal you are preparing.

Some Good Eating Tips

Drink Water

When you are eating, do not forget to drink water. Water supersedes whatever liquid you plan on taking with your meal. Ensure that you drink water before eating because this practice helps your metabolism and fills your stomach. And more importantly, it does not contain calories, artificial sweeteners, and sugar.

Do not Snack After Dinner

Having snacks after dinner is not advisable because eating late at night might lead to acid reflux and negatively affect your blood pressure, blood sugar, and weight. However, if you are still hungry after dinner, you can opt for foods with high protein and fiber and do not consume the food in large portions.

Eat in Smaller Bits

Instead of shoveling a handful of food into your mouth, eat in smaller bits. Eating smaller bites can have several benefits. One reason is that it can help you to eat more slowly, which can lead to better digestion and more enjoyable eating experiences. When you eat more slowly, your body has more time to register that you're full, which can help you eat less overall and potentially improve weight management. Eating smaller bites can also be easier on your digestive system, as the food is more easily broken down and absorbed. It can also be less overwhelming to eat smaller portions at a time, which can be helpful if you're trying to reduce portion sizes or are feeling full.

Healthy Treats or Snacks to Satisfy Your Cravings at Home

Sometimes, even after having our meals, we can still crave something sugary or sweet like ice cream, cookies, or a candy bar. There are other sweeter things you can consume without endangering your health. Healthy snacks can be fresh, frozen, dried fruit, smoothies, chocolates, and treats that are made from whole foods like seeds, nuts, dates, and coconuts.

Some Healthy Snack Tips:

- Understand your body system because sometimes you might not be actually hungry but you might just be in the mood to visit the office vending machine.
- If there is going to be over four hours between meals (lunch and dinner), then it is advisable to eat a snack to avoid getting hungry or overeating in the evening.

- Try as much as possible to minimize or limit added sugars. Added sugars can cause heart disease, weight gain or obesity, and type 2 diabetes. The Centers for Disease Control and Prevention (CDC) recommends that you should limit your intake of added sugar and not take more than ten percent of your daily calories or no more than six added teaspoons per day. Also, if you cannot make your snack at home and you prefer to purchase pre-packaged snacks, check the labels and look out for sneaky sugars like malt syrup, lactose, fructose, corn syrup, corn sweetener, and organic cane juice.

Healthy Treats or Snacks

- Whole grain crackers with avocado spread.
- Baked apples.
- Roasted pumpkin seeds.
- Apple slices with almond butter.
- Hard-boiled eggs.
- Energy balls made with oats, nuts, and dried fruit.
- Dessert hummus with strawberries.
- Baby carrots with hummus.
- Mandarin oranges and Greek yogurt.

- Greek yogurt with berries.

- Roasted chickpeas.

- Tuna salad stuffed into cherry tomatoes.

- Edamame.

- Trail mix with nuts, seeds, and dried fruit.

- Sliced bell peppers with guacamole.

A great tip for saving time in the kitchen is ***Cook once, and eat more than once:*** you do not have to cook every day. You can cook once, and eat the food more than once. This principle will help you to save time and be more efficient in the kitchen which will make it easier for you to stick to your meal plans. This means that you cook twice the quantity you would normally cook the food, and store the excess or remnant in the refrigerator or freezer. How does this save time? Cooking a meal requires so much time and energy, and if you cook several quantities now, you would not have to repeat the process. You can do this by ensuring that there are leftovers from every meal you prepare. The leftovers will be kept in the refrigerator or freezer for future meals. Soups and stews are excellent leftovers. Your leftover meal can also be used to prepare another meal. For example, leftover grilled chicken can be used to make Greek salad wrap.

What Makes a Meal Plan Healthy?

A healthy meal plan gives your body the needed nutrients daily which helps to lower heart and other related diseases. It controls food portions, limits sodium added sugars, and trans fats, includes meats, poultry, beans, and eggs, and focuses on vegetables, fruits, whole grains, and low-fat or fat-free dairy products.

- *Vegetables:* vegetables should be an important part of your diet. The more vegetables you have, the better for you.
- *Fruits:* always include fresh or frozen fruits in your diet.
- *Whole Grains:* whole wheat, oats, barley, and quinoa are great options to incorporate into your meal plan.
- *Nuts and Seeds:* Preferably go for plain nuts. Limit salted or roasted nuts. Avoid nuts containing other flavors like honey because they contain added sugar.
- *Lean Proteins:* go for proteins like turkey, chicken, fish, and legumes.
- *Legumes:* foods high in protein and fiber like beans and lentils.
- *Healthy Fats:* great healthy fat options include salmon, olive oil, and avocado.

How to Design Your Own Meal Plan Template

If you have never created your own meal plan template, do not worry. This section contains a step-by-step guide to help you create the perfect meal plan template.

Meal Chart: the meal chart is usually in the form of a grid. That is, the days of the week will be on one axis, while the type of meal will be on another axis.

	Breakfast	Lunch	Dinner
Monday			
Tuesday			
Wednesday			
Thursday			
Friday			
Saturday			
Sunday			

Budget: if you are working within a budget, you can also include the budget in another column or row.

Meal Plan on a Budget

- Develop a plan. The plan should include creating a list of items that will be needed from the market so that you do not have to spend money on convenience meals or fast foods.

- You can plan your meals around foods that are on sale. You can check newspaper inserts, coupon sites online, or store flyers.

- You can also eat a meatless meal a week. For example, beans and dried peas.

- Eat grains more often. Grains like pasta, rice, and barley are inexpensive and can be cooked in many different ways.

- Do not go for recipes that require special or expensive ingredients. If you must purchase such ingredients, ask questions such as, is the package big or small? Can you use it up before it expires? Is it worth the money?

- Do not throw away leftovers.

- Cook in bulk by making extras. For example, do not let a big bunch of carrots go to waste, instead, you can use it to make an extra big pot of soup.

- Know what everyone in the family likes to eat to avoid wastage.

28-Days Meal Plan

WEEK 1

SHOPPING LIST

Banana Yogurt Pots

- 2 bananas.

- 15g tablespoons of walnuts.

- Greek yogurt.

White Bean-Tomato Toast

- Whole wheat bread.

- 1/15 oz. can of white beans, drained and rinsed.

- Extra-virgin olive oil.

- 1 lemon.

- Salt and pepper.

- 5 cherry tomatoes.

Green Smoothie

- Fresh baby spinach or frozen baby spinach.
- Fresh or frozen blueberries.
- Chia seeds.
- 1 cup of almond milk.

Avocado Spread

- 2 peeled, pitted, and chopped avocados.
- Black pepper.
- Lime juice.
- Olive oil.
- Salt.
- Shallots.
- Coconut cream.
- Chopped chives.

Tomato and Watermelon Salad

- Olive oil.
- Red wine vinegar.

- Chilli flakes.

- Mint.

- Tomatoes.

- Watermelon.

- Feta cheese.

Spinach Omelet

- Black pepper.

- Baby spinach.

- Olive oil.

- 8 Eggs.

- Sweet paprika.

- 2 onions.

- Ground cumin.

- Chives.

White Bean-Tomato Spread

- Whole wheat bread.

- White beans.

- Extra-virgin olive oil.

- 1 lemon.
- Salt and pepper.
- 5 cherry tomatoes.

Pita Slaw Sandwich

- Whole wheat pita.
- 2 cups mixed greens, broccoli slaw, and romaine lettuce.
- 4 Sundried tomatoes.
- Green-ball pepper.
- Store-bought hummus.
- 1 hard-boiled egg (optional).

Cannellini Bean Salad

- Cannellini beans
- Cherry tomatoes, halved
- Red onion.
- Red wine vinegar
- Small bunch of basil.

Blueberry, Peach, and Avocado Spread

- Extra virgin olive oil.
- Lime juice.
- Lime zest.
- Teaspoon salt.
- 2 blueberries.
- 1 avocado.
- 2 large ripe peaches.
- Fresh basil.

Turkey-Ginger Sliders

- Lean turkey.
- Ginger.
- Shallot.
- Tomato paste.
- Salt and pepper.
- Extra-virgin olive oil.
- Medium cucumber.
- Whole grain slider buns.

Garlicky Kale and Pea Sauté

- 2 garlic cloves.
- 1 hot red chili.
- Olive oil.
- 2 bunches of kale.
- 1 lb. frozen peas.

Edgy Veggie Wraps

- 100g cherry tomato.
- 1 cucumber.
- 6 kalamata olives.
- 2 large wholemeal tortilla wraps.
- 50g / ¼ cup feta cheese.
- Hummus

Chicken Thighs and Grapes Mix

- Garlic cloves.
- Tomatoes.
- Yellow onion.

- Black pepper.

- Chicken stock, low-sodium.

- Chicken thighs.

- Carrot.

- Olive oil.

- Green grapes.

Five-Spice Chicken Breast

- Black pepper.

- Five-spice.

- Hot pepper.

- Avocado oil.

- Cilantro.

- Chicken breast.

- Tomatoes.

- Coconut aminos.

Almond-Crusted Baked Salmon

- Dijon mustard.

- 1 lemon zest.

- Herbs of choice (dill, lemon thyme, chives, parsley).

- 4/6 oz. thick-cut salmon fillets.

- Pepper.

- Almonds.

Salmon with Potatoes and Corn Salad

- 200g baby new potatoes

- 1 sweetcorn cob

- 2 skinless salmon fillets

- 60g tomatoes

- Red wine vinegar.

- Extra-virgin olive oil.

- Bunch of spring onions/scallions.

- Capers.

- A handful of basil leaves.

Walnut Salmon Mix

- 4 salmon fillets.

- Avocado oil.

- Salt.

- Black pepper.
- Lime juice.
- Shallots.
- Walnuts.
- Parsley.

Salmon and Tomatoes

- Avocado oil.
- Salmon fillets.
- Cherry tomatoes.
- Spring onions.
- Vegetable stock.
- Salt and black pepper.
- Dried rosemary.

	BREAKFAST	LUNCH	DINNER
MONDAY	White bean-tomato toast	Pita slaw sandwich	Chicken thighs and grapes mix
TUESDAY	Green smoothie	Cannellini bean salad	Five-spice chicken breast
WEDNESDAY	Avocado Spread	Blueberry, peach, and avocado spread	Almond-crusted baked salmon
THURSDAY	Blueberry-coconut overnight spread	Turkey-Ginger sliders	Salmon with potatoes and corn salad
FRIDAY	Tomato and watermelon salad	Garlicky kale and pea sauté	Walnut salmon mix
SATURDAY	Spinach omelet	Edgy veggie wraps	Salmon and Tomatoes
SUNDAY	White bean-tomato spread	Pita slaw sandwich	Spicy tomato baked egg

WEEK 2

SHOPPING LIST

White Bean-Tomato Toast

- Whole wheat bread.
- 1/15 oz. can of white beans, drained and rinsed.
- Extra-virgin olive oil.
- 1 lemon.
- Salt and pepper.
- 5 cherry tomatoes.

Pita Slaw Sandwich

- Whole wheat pita.
- 2 cups mixed greens, broccoli slaw, and romaine lettuce.
- 4 Sundried tomatoes.
- Green-ball pepper.
- Store-bought hummus.
- 1 hard-boiled egg (optional).

Chicken Thighs and Grapes Mix

- Garlic cloves.

- Tomatoes.

- Yellow onion.

- Black pepper.

- Chicken stock, low-sodium.

- Chicken thighs.

- Carrot.

- Olive oil.

- Green grapes.

Green Smoothie

- Fresh baby spinach or frozen baby spinach.

- Fresh or frozen blueberries.

- Chia seeds.

- 1 cup of almond milk.

Cannellini Bean Salad

- Cannellini beans

- Cherry tomatoes, halved
- Red onion.
- Red wine vinegar
- Small bunch of basil.

Five-Spice Chicken Breast

- Black pepper.
- Five-spice.
- Hot pepper.
- Avocado oil.
- Cilantro.
- Chicken breast.
- Tomatoes.
- Coconut aminos.

Avocado Spread

- 2 peeled, pitted, and chopped avocados.
- Black pepper.
- Lime juice.
- Olive oil.

- Salt.

- Shallots.

- Coconut cream.

- Chopped chives.

Blueberry, Peach, And Avocado Spread

- Extra virgin olive oil.

- Lime juice.

- Lime zest.

- Teaspoon salt.

- 2 blueberries.

- 1 avocado.

- 2 large ripe peaches.

- Fresh basil.

Tomato and Watermelon Salad

- Olive oil.

- Red wine vinegar.

- Chilli flakes.

- Mint.

- Tomatoes.

- Watermelon.

- Feta cheese.

Turkey-Ginger Sliders

- Lean turkey.

- Ginger.

- Shallot.

- Tomato paste.

- Salt and pepper.

- Extra-virgin olive oil.

- Medium cucumber.

- Whole grain slider buns.

Salmon with Potatoes and Corn Salad

- 200g baby new potatoes

- 1 sweetcorn cob

- 2 skinless salmon fillets

- 60g tomatoes

- Red wine vinegar.

- Extra-virgin olive oil.

- Bunch of spring onions/scallions.

- Capers.

- A handful of basil leaves.

Garlicky Kale and Pea Sauté

- 2 garlic cloves.

- 1 hot red chili.

- Olive oil.

- 2 bunches of kale.

- 1 lb. frozen peas.

Walnut Salmon Mix

- 4 salmon fillets.

- Avocado oil.

- Salt.

- Black pepper.

- Lime juice.

- Shallots.

- Walnuts.

- Parsley.

Spinach Omelet

- Black pepper.
- Baby spinach.
- Olive oil.
- 8 Eggs.
- Sweet paprika.
- 2 onions.
- Ground cumin.
- Chives.

Edgy Veggie Wraps

- 100g cherry tomato.
- 1 cucumber.
- 6 kalamata olives.
- 2 large wholemeal tortilla wraps.
- 50g / ¼ cup feta cheese.
- Hummus.

Salmon and Tomatoes

- Avocado oil.

- Salmon fillets.

- Cherry tomatoes.

- Spring onions.

- Vegetable stock.

- Salt and black pepper.

- Dried rosemary.

	BREAKFAST	**LUNCH**	**DINNER**
MONDAY	Banana yogurt pots	Rice and bean burritos	Moussaka
TUESDAY	Avocado toast	Pistachio-crusted trout	Spicy tomato baked egg
WEDNESDAY	Tomato and watermelon salad	Flavorful refried beans	Black bean stuffed sweet potato
THURSDAY	Blueberry oats bowl	Chicken, tomato, and spinach salad	Salmon and Tomatoes
FRIDAY	Green smoothie	Edgy veggie wraps	Five-spice chicken breast
SATURDAY	Polenta with a dose of cranberries and pears	Blueberry, peach, and avocado spread	Cauliflower steak with sweat-pea puree
SUNDAY	One egg wonder	Cannellini bean salad	Chicken thighs and grapes mix

WEEK 3

SHOPPING LIST

Spinach Omelet

- Black pepper.
- Baby spinach.
- Olive oil.
- 8 Eggs.
- Sweet paprika.
- 2 onions.
- Ground cumin.
- Chives.

One-Egg Wonder

- Egg.
- 3 heirloom cherry tomatoes, halved.
- Extra-virgin olive oil.
- Salt and pepper.

Avocado Spread

- 2 peeled, pitted, and chopped avocados.
- Black pepper.
- Lime juice.
- Olive oil.
- Salt.
- Shallots.
- Coconut cream.
- Chopped chives.

Blueberry-Coconut Overnight Oats

- Frozen blueberries.
- Banana.
- Plain Greek yogurt.
- Cup of water.
- Rolled oats.
- Unsweetened shredded coconut.

Creamy Berry Smoothie

- Fresh or frozen blueberries.
- Fresh or frozen strawberries.
- Soft, drained tofu.
- Unsweetened almond-coconut milk blend.
- Almond butter.

Banana Yogurt Pots

- 2 bananas.
- 15g of walnuts.
- Greek yogurt.

Avocado Toast

- Whole wheat bread.
- Avocado.
- Red onions.
- Extra virgin olive oil.
- Salt and pepper.
- Lemon.

- Chilli pepper flakes.

Chickpea and Spinach Cutlets

- Red bell pepper.
- 19 ounces of chickpeas.
- Ground almonds.
- Dijon mustard.
- Oregano.
- Sage.
- Fresh spinach.
- Rolled oats.
- Garlic.
- Lemon.
- Pure maple syrup.

Chicken, Tomato, and Spinach Salad

- Chopped red onion.
- Black pepper.
- Baby spinach.
- Rotisserie chicken.

- Cherry tomatoes.

- Green pea.

- Lemon juice.

- Walnuts.

- Olive oil.

Edgy Veggie Wraps

- 100g cherry tomato.

- 1 cucumber.

- 6 kalamata olives.

- 2 large wholemeal tortilla wraps.

- 50g / ¼ cup feta cheese.

- Hummus.

Rice and Bean Burritos

- Tortillas.

- Fat-free refried beans.

- Rice.

- Olive oil.

- Salsa.

- Green onions.

- Bell peppers.

- Guacamole

Flavorful Refried Beans

- Pinto beans.

- Jalapeno pepper.

- White onion.

- Garlic.

- Salt.

- Black pepper.

- Ground cumin.

- Water.

Pita Slaw Sandwich

- Whole wheat pita.

- Greens, broccoli slaw, and romaine lettuce.

- Sundried tomatoes.

- Green-ball pepper.

- Store-bought hummus.

- Egg (optional).

Garlicky Kale and Pea Sauté

- Garlic cloves.
- Red Chilli.
- Olive oil.
- Kale.
- Frozen peas.

Black Bean Stuffed Sweet Potato

- Sweet potatoes.
- Black beans.
- Black pepper.
- Red onion.
- Sea salt.
- Onion powder.
- Garlic powder.
- Red chili powder.
- Cumin.
- Lime juice.

- Olive oil.

- Cashew cream sauce.

Salmon with Potatoes and Corn Salad

- Baby new potatoes

- Sweetcorn cob

- Skinless salmon fillets

- Tomatoes

- Red wine vinegar.

- Extra-virgin olive oil.

- Bunch of spring onions/scallions.

- Capers.

- Handful of basil leaves.

Moussaka

- Olive oil

- Onion.

- Garlic clove.

- Lean beef mince

- Tomatoes

- Tomato purée

- Ground cinnamon

- Chickpeas

- Feta cheese

- Dried mint

- Brown bread

Five-Spice Chicken Breast

- Black pepper.

- Five-spice.

- Hot pepper.

- Avocado oil.

- Cilantro.

- Chicken breast halves.

- Tomatoes.

- Coconut aminos.

Almond-crusted Baked Salmon

- Dijon mustard.

- Lemon.

- Herbs of choice (dill, lemon thyme, chives, parsley).

- Salmon fillets.

- Pepper.

- Almonds.

Spicy Tomato Baked Egg

- Olive oil.

- Red onions.

- Red chili.

- Garlic clove.

- Small bunch of coriander.

- Cherry tomatoes

- Eggs.

- Brown bread

	BREAKFAST	LUNCH	DINNER
MONDAY	Spinach omelet	Chickpea and spinach cutlets	Black bean stuffed sweet potato
TUESDAY	One egg wonder	Chicken, tomato, and spinach salad	Salmon with potatoes and corn salad
WEDNESDAY	Avocado spread	Edgy veggie wraps	Moussaka
THURSDAY	Blueberry-coconut overnight oats	Rice and bean burritos	Five-spice chicken breast
FRIDAY	Creamy berry smoothie	Flavorful refried beans	Almond-crusted baked salmon
SATURDAY	Banana yogurt pot	Pita slaw sandwich	Moussaka
SUNDAY	Avocado toast	Garlicky kale and pea sauté	Spicy tomato baked egg

WEEK 4

SHOPPING LIST

Banana Yogurt Pots

- Bananas.
- Walnuts.
- Greek yogurt.

Spinach Omelet

- Black pepper.
- Baby spinach.
- Olive oil.
- Eggs.
- Sweet paprika.
- Onions.
- Ground cumin.
- Chives.

White Bean-Tomato Spread

- Whole wheat bread.

- White beans.

- Extra-virgin olive oil.

- Lemon.

- Salt and pepper.

- Cherry tomatoes.

Tomato and Watermelon Salad

- Olive oil.

- Red wine vinegar.

- Chilli flakes.

- Mint.

- Tomatoes.

- Watermelon.

- Feta cheese.

One-Egg Wonder

- Egg.

- Heirloom cherry tomatoes, halved.
- Extra-virgin olive oil.
- Salt and pepper.

Polenta with a Dose of Cranberries and Pears

- Freshly cored pears.
- Warm basic polenta.
- Brown rice syrup.
- Cinnamon, ground.
- Fresh cranberries

Creamy Berry Smoothie

- Fresh or frozen blueberries.
- Fresh or frozen strawberries.
- Soft, drained tofu.
- Unsweetened almond-coconut milk blend.
- Almond butter.

Pita Slaw Sandwich

- Whole wheat pita.
- Mixed greens, broccoli slaw, and romaine lettuce.
- Sundried tomatoes.
- Green-bell pepper.
- Store-bought hummus.
- Egg (optional).

Turkey-Ginger Sliders

- Lean turkey.
- Ginger.
- Shallot.
- Tomato paste.
- Salt and pepper.
- Extra-virgin olive oil.
- Medium size cucumber.
- Whole grain slider buns.

Blueberry, Peach, and Avocado Spread

- Extra-virgin olive oil.
- Lime juice.
- Lime zest.
- Salt.
- Blueberries.
- Avocado.
- Peaches.
- Fresh basil.

Cannellini Bean Salad

- Cannellini beans
- Cherry tomatoes halved
- Red onion.
- Red wine vinegar
- Small bunch of basil.

Pistachio-Crusted Trout

- Trout fillets.

- Fresh lemon.

- Salt.

- Pepper.

- Shelled pistachios.

Rice and Bean Burritos

- Tortillas.

- Fat-free refried beans.

- Rice.

- Olive oil.

- Salsa

- Green onions, chopped.

- Bell peppers, chopped.

- Guacamole

Flavorful Refried Beans

- Pinto beans.

- Seeded jalapeno pepper, chopped.

- White onion, peeled.

- Minced garlic.

- Salt.

- Ground black pepper.

- Ground cumin.

Chicken Thighs and Grapes Mix

- Garlic cloves.

- Tomatoes.

- Yellow onion.

- Black pepper.

- Chicken stock, low-sodium.

- Chicken thighs.

- Carrot.

- Olive oil.

- Green grapes.

Salmon and Tomatoes

- Avocado oil.

- Salmon fillets.

- Cherry tomatoes.

- Spring onions.

- Vegetable stock.

- Salt and black pepper.

- Dried rosemary.

Five-Spice Chicken Breast

- Black pepper.

- Five-spice.

- Hot pepper.

- Avocado oil.

- Cilantro.

- Chicken breast.

- Tomatoes.

- Coconut aminos.

Black Bean Stuffed Sweet Potato

- Sweet potatoes.

- Black beans.

- Ground black pepper.

- Red onion, peeled and diced.

- Sea salt.

- Onion powder.

- Garlic powder.

- Red chili powder.

- Cumin.

- Lime juice.

- Olive oil.

- Cashew cream sauce.

Cauliflower Steak with Sweet-Pea Puree

- Cauliflower.

- Olive oil.

- Paprika.

- Coriander.

- Black pepper sweet-pea puree.

- Frozen green peas.

- Onion.

- Fresh parsley.

- Unsweetened soy milk.

Spicy Tomato Baked Egg

- Olive oil.

- Red onions.

- Red chili.

- Garlic clove.

- Small bunch of coriander.

- Cherry tomatoes.

- Eggs.

- Brown bread.

	BREAKFAST	**LUNCH**	**DINNER**
MONDAY	Polenta with a dose of cranberries and pears.	Flavorful refried beans	Chicken thighs and grape mix
TUESDAY	White bean tomato spread	Pita slaw sandwich	Black bean stuffed sweet potato
WEDNESDAY	Creamy berry smoothie	Turkey-ginger sliders	Salmon and tomato
THURSDAY	One egg wonder	Rice and bean burritos	Cauliflower steak with sweet pea puree
FRIDAY	Banana yogurt pots	Blueberry, peach, and avocado spread	Spicy tomato baked egg
SATURDAY	Tomato and watermelon salad	Pistachio-crusted trout	Salmon and tomato
SUNDAY	Spinach omelet	Cannellini bean salad	Five-spice chicken breast

BOOK 3

IVAN BURROWS

BREAKFAST RECIPES

Green Smoothie

The MIND diet recommends eating lots of leafy greens in your diet, and the green smoothie is a great way of adding leafy greens to your everyday diet.

It contains 8g of fat, 33g of carbohydrates, 5g of protein, and 210 calories.

Time: 5 minutes

Servings: 1 serving

Ingredients:

- 1 cup of fresh baby spinach or ½ cup of frozen baby spinach
- 1 cup of fresh or frozen blueberries
- 1 tablespoon of chia seeds
- 1 cup of almond milk

Direction:

Mix all the ingredients in a blender, and blend them until you get a smooth and thick consistency.

Spinach Omelet

It contains 12g of fat, 8g of carbohydrates, 13.3g of protein, and 345 calories.

Time: 20 minutes

Servings: 4 servings

Ingredients:

- black pepper
- 1 cup of baby spinach
- 1 tablespoon of olive oil
- 8 whisked eggs
- 1 tablespoon of sweet paprika
- 2 chopped spring onions
- 1 tablespoon of ground cumin
- 1 tablespoon of chopped chives

Direction:

Heat the pan, and add the spring onions, paprika, and cumin. Stir the mixture and allow it to sauté for 5 minutes. Then, add the eggs, spinach, pepper into the pan, and cover it, and allow it to cook for about 14 minutes. Then, sprinkle the chives on top and serve.

Avocado Spread

Avocado is a great source of unsaturated fats, which contain several nutrients that are good for the brain as they help to lower cognitive decline.

It contains 0.5g of fat, 15g of carbohydrates, 1g of protein, and 79 calories.

Time: 1 minute

Servings: 4 servings

Ingredients:

- 2 peeled, pitted, and chopped avocados
- black pepper
- 1 tablespoon of lime juice
- 1 tablespoon of olive oil
- salt
- 1 tablespoon of minced shallots
- 1 tablespoon of heavy coconut cream
- 1 tablespoon of chopped chives

Direction:

Put the avocado flesh, oil, shallots, and the other ingredients except for the chives into the blender. Blend properly, then pour into bowls, sprinkle chives on the top, and serve with whole-grain bread.

Avocado Toast

It contains 8g of fat, 16g of carbohydrates 4g of protein, and 150 calories.

Time: 5 minutes

Servings: 4 servings

Ingredients:

- 4 slices of whole wheat bread
- 1 peeled, deseeded, and mashed avocado
- thinly sliced ½ small red onions
- 2 teaspoons of extra virgin olive oil
- salt and pepper
- 1 lemon, quartered
- ½ teaspoon of chili pepper flakes

Direction:

Toast the bread to your desired taste. Evenly distribute the mashed avocado on the four slices of whole wheat bread. Add red onions to the mashed avocados, drizzle olive oil on them, and sprinkle chilly pepper flakes, salt, and pepper. Squeeze lemon on the avocado toast before eating.

Creamy Berry Smoothie

Berries are high in flavonoids, and they improve cognition.

It contains 8g of fat, 24g of carbohydrates, 6g of protein, and 180 calories.

Time: 5 minutes

Servings: 2 servings

Ingredients:

- 1 cup of fresh or frozen blueberries
- 1 cup of fresh or frozen strawberries
- ½ cup of soft, drained tofu
- ½ cup of unsweetened almond-coconut milk blend
- 1 tablespoon of almond butter

Direction:

Put all the ingredients in the blender, and blend till it is fully combined.

Almond Quinoa

It contains 21g of fat, 40g of carbohydrates, 8g of protein, and 380 calories.

Time: 12 minutes

Servings: 2 servings

Ingredients:

- ¾ cup of quinoa, soaked in water for at least 1 hour
- ¾ cup of water
- 8 ounces of almond milk
- ½ tablespoon of crushed almonds
- 2 tablespoons of honey
- 1 tablespoon of vanilla extract
- 1 pinch of salt toppings
- ¼ cup of soaked, peeled, and chopped almonds

Direction:

Put all the ingredients in an instant pot and press the rice function key. Put the time to ten minutes and press cook at low pressure. When it is cooked, pour it into the bowl and add almonds on top.

Banana Yogurt Pots

It contains 7g of fat, 54g of carbohydrates, 20g of protein, and 302 calories.

Time: 5 minutes

Servings: 2servings

Ingredients:

- 2 bananas, sliced into chunks.
- 2 tablespoons of walnuts, toasted and chopped.
- 1 cup Greek yogurt.

Direction:

Pour some yogurt into the bottom of a glass. Add a layer of banana, then yogurt, then banana, and repeat until the glass is full. Then, scatter with nuts.

White Bean-Tomato Toast

It contains 8g of fat, 27g of carbohydrates, 8g of protein, and 200 calories.

Time: 5 minutes

Servings: 1 serving

Ingredients:

- 1 slice/of 100% whole wheat bread.
- 1/15 oz. can of white beans, drained and rinsed.
- 4 teaspoons of extra-virgin olive oil, divided.
- 1 lemon, juiced.
- salt and pepper, to taste.
- 5 cherry tomatoes, halved.

Direction:

Place your bread in the toaster. Meanwhile, blend beans, lemon juice, 3 teaspoons of olive oils, and salt and pepper until uniform. It should have a spread-like consistency like hummus. You can add more olive oil to get the desired consistency. Spread 2 tablespoons of the white beans mixture onto the toast, top with halved tomatoes, and drizzle with the remaining teaspoon of olive oil. Season with extra pepper as desired. There will be leftover spread which can be kept in the fridge and eaten for up to five days. This recipe can be repeated or the spread can be enjoyed as a dip in an easy snack with strips of carrots, celery, cucumbers, or bell peppers.

Blueberry-Coconut Overnight Oats

It contains 5g of fat, 43g of carbohydrates, 15g of protein, and 270 calories.

Time: 5 minutes to prepare and 5+ hours refrigeration

Servings: 2 servings

Ingredients:

- ¾ cup of frozen blueberries.
- ½ banana.
- ¾ cup of plain Greek yogurt.
- ½ cup of water.
- ¾ cup of rolled oats.
- 3 tablespoons of unsweetened shredded coconut.

Direction:

Put the blueberries, banana, yogurt, and water in a blender and blend until smooth. Pour the mixture into a bowl. Mix in the oats and coconuts. Separate the mixture into 2 separate containers and cover them with a lid. Refrigerate for at least 5 hours or overnight.

Blueberry Oats Bowl

It contains 4g of fat, 38g of carbohydrates, 13g of protein, and 235 calories.

Time: 5 minutes to prepare and 5 minutes to cook

Servings: 2 servings

Ingredients:

- ⅔ cup porridge oats
- ⅗ cup Greek yogurt
- 1 ¾ cups blueberries
- 1 teaspoon honey

Direction:

Pour 400ml of water into a pan, and pour oats in it. Heat and stir for about 2 minutes, then, remove heat and pour a third of the yogurt. Tip the blueberries into a pan with honey and add 1 tablespoon of water. Then, gently poach it until the blueberries are tender. Spoon the porridge into bowls and add the remaining blueberries and yogurt.

Tomato and Watermelon Salad

It contains 13g of fat, 13g of carbohydrates, 5g of protein, and 175 calories.

Time: 5 minutes

Servings: 2 servings

Ingredients:

- 1 tablespoon of olive oil
- 1 tablespoon of red wine vinegar
- ¼ teaspoon of chili flakes
- 1 tablespoon of chopped mint
- ½ cup of tomatoes, chopped
- ½ watermelon, cut into chunks
- ⅔ cup feta cheese, crumbled.

Direction:

For the dressing, mix the oil, vinegar, chili flakes, and mint, then season. Pour the tomatoes and watermelon into a bowl. Pour over the dressing, add the feta, and serve.

One-Egg Wonder

It contains 1g of fat, 2g of carbohydrates, 7g of protein, and 120 calories.

Time: 5 minutes

Servings: 2 servings

Ingredients:

- 1 egg
- 3 heirloom cherry tomatoes, halved
- 1 teaspoon of extra-virgin olive oil
- salt and pepper, to taste.

Direction:

Crack the egg into a 4-to-6 oz. ramekin. Beat the egg with a fork to incorporate a lot of air which will result in a fluffier cooked egg. Microwave for about 45 to 60 seconds. Remove carefully from the microwave as the ramekin will be hot. Top it with tomato halves and drizzle with olive.

Polenta with a Dose of Cranberries and Pears

It contains 5g of fat, 6g of carbohydrates, 5g of protein, and 185 calories.

Time: 12 minutes

Servings: 4 servings

Ingredients:

- 2 freshly cored pears, peeled and diced
- 1 batch of warm basic polenta
- ¼ cup of brown rice syrup
- 1 teaspoon of cinnamon, ground
- 1 cup of fresh cranberries

Direction:

Pour the polenta into a saucepan and warm. Then, stir in pears, cinnamon powder, and cranberries. Cook until the pears become soft in 10 minutes. Divide into 4 bowls. Top with some pear compote.

LUNCH RECIPES

Rice and Bean Burritos

It contains 6g of fat, 49g of carbohydrates, 9g of protein, and 290 calories.

Time: 20 minutes

Servings: 8 servings

Ingredients:

- 6 tortillas
- 32 ounces of fat-free refried beans
- 2 cups of cooked rice
- 1 tablespoon of olive oil
- ½ cup of salsa
- 1 bunch of green onions, chopped
- 2 bell peppers, chopped
- Guacamole

Direction:

Preheat the oven to 375°F. Then, put the refried beans into a saucepan and place over medium heat to warm. Heat the tortillas and lay them out on a flat surface. Spoon the beans into a long mound that runs across the tortilla, just from the center. Next, spoon some rice and salsa on the beans and add the onions, green peppers, and chopped vegetables (optional) to taste. Fold over the shortest edge of the plain tortilla roll it up, and fold in the sides as you go. Put each burrito, seam side down, on a nonstick-sprayed baking sheet. Brush with olive oil and bake for 15 minutes, then serve with guacamole.

Chicken, Tomato, and Spinach Salad

It contains 40g of fat, 1g of carbohydrates, 17g of protein, and 380 calories.

Time: 3 minutes

Servings: 4 servings

Ingredients:

- 1 chopped red onion
- ½ tablespoon of black pepper
- 4 cups of baby spinach
- 2 de-boned, skinless, and shredded rotisserie chicken
- 1 lb. halved cherry tomatoes
- green pea
- 2 tablespoons of lemon juice
- ¼ cup of chopped walnuts
- 1 tablespoon of olive oil

Direction:

Combine all the ingredients in a salad bowl, toss, and serve for lunch.

Pita Slaw Sandwich

It contains 5g of fat, 28g of carbohydrates, 11g of protein, and 190 calories.

Time: 5 minutes and 15 minutes for the hard-boiling egg

Servings: 2 servings

Ingredients:

- 1 whole wheat pita
- 2 cups mixed greens, broccoli slaw, and romaine lettuce
- 4 pieces of sundried tomatoes
- 2 teaspoons of green-ball pepper
- 2 tablespoons of store-bought hummus
- 1 hard-boiled egg (optional)

Direction:

Cut the pita into half and place it in a toaster if you want it to be slightly crunchy. Add 1 cup of lettuce mix and 1 teaspoon of green-ball pepper to each pita half. Add 2 pieces of sun-dried tomatoes, a tablespoon of hummus, and half of the hard-boiled egg (optional) to each half. Prewashed broccoli slaw is best for this recipe.

Curried Chickpea Quinoa Loaf

It contains 9g of fat, 44g of carbohydrates, 12g of protein, and 300 calories.

Time: 2 hours and 10 minutes

Servings: 6 servings

Ingredients:

- 1 teaspoon of extra virgin olive oil
- 1 onion, diced
- 1 fresh turmeric root or 1 teaspoon of dried turmeric
- 1-½ teaspoon garam masala, divided
- ½ teaspoon of plus pinch cumin, divided
- ¼ teaspoon plus a pinch of red chili flakes, divided
- 2 cloves garlic, minced
- 1 teaspoon minced ginger
- pinch sea salt (optional)
- 1 cup of diced mushrooms
- 1 cup of chopped fresh greens (for example spinach, chard, and kale)
- 2 tablespoons and 1 teaspoon of fresh, chopped parsley

- 1-½ cups of tomato sauce, divided

- 2 tablespoons of chia seeds

- 2 cups of cooked quinoa

- 1 cup of cooked or canned chickpeas, mashed slightly

- 1/3 cup of chopped cashews

- ½ cup of dry oats

Direction:

Heat the oil in a skillet under medium heat, and sauté the onion for two minutes. Add turmeric root, 1 teaspoon of garam masala, ½ teaspoon of cumin, ¼ teaspoon of red chili flakes, garlic, ginger, and salt (optional), and sauté for 1 minute. Then, add mushrooms, greens, and parsley, and sauté for 2 minutes.

Transfer the onion mixtures into a large bowl. In a separate medium bowl, mix ½ cup of tomato sauce with chia seeds, and allow to stand for five minutes. Also, add quinoa, chickpeas, cashews, and oats to the onion mixture and combine them well.

Spray a loaf pan with nonstick cooking spray and transfer the mixture to the pan. Press the content into the pan firmly. Put in the refrigerator and let it chill for 1 hour. Next, preheat the oven to 350°F and bake for 50 minutes until golden and firm. Let it cool before slicing it into thick slices.

Mix 1 cup of tomato sauce with the remaining pinch of turmeric, ½ teaspoon of garam masala, a pinch of cumin, and a pinch of red chili flakes, and heat in a small pot until warm enough. Then, serve each loaf slice with a ladle of tomato sauce.

Chickpea and Spinach Cutlets

It contains 11g of fat, 21g of carbohydrates, 8g of protein, and 200 calories.

Time: 40 minutes

Servings: 12 servings

Ingredients:

- 1 red bell pepper
- 19 ounces of chickpeas, rinsed and drained
- 1 cup of ground almonds
- 2 teaspoons of Dijon mustard
- 1 teaspoon of oregano
- ½ teaspoon of sage
- 1 cup of fresh spinach
- 1½ cups of rolled oats
- 1 clove of garlic, pressed
- ½ lemon, juiced
- 2 teaspoons of pure maple syrup

Direction:

Line a baking sheet with parchment paper. Then, cut the red bell pepper in half and remove the seeds. Put it on the baking sheet and roast it in the oven. Process your chickpeas, mustard, almonds, and maple syrup together in a food processor. Add your lemon juice, sage, oregano, garlic, and spinach, and process it again. Make sure it is combined but do not puree it. Your red bell pepper should take about ten minutes to become softened, then add it to the processor as well. Also, add your oats and mix them very well. After that, form twelve patties and cook in the oven for half an hour until browned.

Roasted Chicken with Fennel, Carrots, and Dried Plums

It contains 12g of fat, 19g of carbohydrates, 54g of protein, and 420 calories.

Time: 1 hour 25 minutes

Servings: 8 to 10 servings

Ingredients:

- 1 pound of carrots, peeled, halved lengthwise, and cut into ½ inch chunks (about 3 cups)
- 1 large fennel bulb, sliced (about 3 cups)
- 2 onions, sliced into half-moons
- 3 tablespoons of extra-virgin olive oil, divided
- 1 tablespoon of chopped fresh rosemary (or 1 teaspoon, dried)
- 1 teaspoon of dried marjoram
- 1 teaspoon of chili powder
- 2 whole-bone in chicken breasts (or 4 split bone-in chicken breasts)
- 1 tablespoon of lemon juice
- 2 cloves of garlic, chopped

- ¾ cup of dry white wine or low-sodium chicken broth, divided
- salt and pepper, to taste
- 1 cup of dried plums, chopped

Direction:

Preheat your oven to 400°F. Then, spread your carrots, fennel, and onions on the bottom of the large roasting pan. Toss it with t tablespoon of olive oil.

Whisk the remaining tablespoons of olive oil with the rosemary, marjoram, and chili powder to form a paste. Then, spread the paste on the chicken breast and be sure to get under the skin. Put it on a roasting rack over the vegetables. Drizzle lemon juice over the chicken breasts and sprinkle it with chopped garlic.

Pour ½ cup of wine or broth around the chicken, and not on top. Then sprinkle the chicken and vegetables with salt and pepper. Roast the chicken and vegetables for 35 minutes.

Baste the top of the chicken, toss in prunes, and cook for another 15 to 20 minutes until the chicken skin is nicely browned and the internal temperature is 150°F. Then, let the chicken rest.

If the vegetables need to cook longer, then transfer the chicken to a cutting board to rest, and continue roasting the vegetables for about 5 to 10 minutes. Pour pan drippings into the saucepan. Then, add the remaining ¼ cup of wine or broth. Simmer for 5 to 10 minutes until the gravy reduces.

To serve, slice the chicken off the bone and serve with vegetables/dried plum mixture with gravel on top.

NOTE: Food safety recommendations for chicken is an internal temperature of 165°F. However, chicken continues cooking after being removed from the oven, so to retain moisture, remove it at 150°F.

Flavorful Refried Beans

It contains 1g of fat, 36g of carbohydrates, 13g of protein, and 105 calories.

Time: 6 hours

Servings: 8 servings

Ingredients:

- 3 cups of rinsed pinto beans
- 1 seeded jalapeno pepper, chopped
- 1 sliced white onion, peeled
- 2 tablespoons of minced garlic
- 5 teaspoons of salt
- 2 tablespoons of ground black pepper
- ¼ tablespoons of ground cumin
- 9 cups of water.

Direction:

Put all the ingredients in a 6-quart slow cooker, and stir until it mixes properly. Cover the top, plug in the slow cooker, adjust the cooking time to 6 hours, and allow it to cook on high settings. Add more water if the beans get too dry. Drain and reserve the bean's water when it is cooked. Mash the beans with a potato masher, and pour in the reserved cooking liquid until it reaches your desired mixture. Serve immediately.

Cannellini Bean Salad

It contains 1g of fat, 54g of carbohydrates, 20g of protein, and 302 calories.

Time: 5 minutes

Servings: 2 servings

Ingredients:

- 3 cups cannellini beans
- ⅜ cup cherry tomatoes, halved
- ½ red onion, thinly sliced
- ½ tablespoon red wine vinegar
- small bunch of basil, torn

Direction:

Rinse and drain the beans and mix with the tomatoes, onion, and vinegar. Season, then add basil just before serving.

Turkey-Ginger Sliders

It contains 5g of fat, 33g of carbohydrates, 25g of protein, and 350 calories.

Time: 30 minutes

Servings: 6 sliders

Ingredients:

- 10 oz./95% lean turkey.
- 1/1-inch piece ginger, minced.
- 1 shallot, minced.
- 1 tablespoon of tomato paste
- salt and pepper to taste.
- 2 teaspoons extra-virgin olive oil.
- 1 medium cucumber, sliced on the diagonal.
- 6 whole-grain slider buns.

Direction:

Combine the ground turkey, ginger, shallot, and tomato paste in a medium-sized bowl. Season with salt and pepper. Also, do not forget to wear gloves to mix until combined. Then, form six patties which are about ¼ inch thick. Heat olive oil in a pan on medium-high heat until hot. Add the patties and cook for 1 to 2 minutes per side until cooked through. Transfer to a paper towel-lined plate to drain. Arrange the sliders by placing cucumber slices and patties between buns.

Edgy Veggie Wraps

It contains 11g of fat, 39g of carbohydrates, 11g of protein, and 310 calories.

Time: 10 minutes

Servings: 2 servings

Ingredients:

- ½ cup cherry tomato
- 1 cucumber
- 6 kalamata olives
- 2 large wholemeal tortilla wraps
- ¼ cup feta cheese
- 2 tablespoons of hummus

Direction:

Chop your tomatoes, cut your cucumber into sticks, split the olives, and take out the stones. Then, heat the tortillas. Spread the hummus over the wrap. Put the vegetable mix in the middle and roll it up.

Pistachio-Crusted Trout

It contains 18g of fat, 9g of carbohydrates, 23g of protein, and 280 calories.

Time: 30 minutes

Servings: 4 servings

Ingredients:

- 4/6-8 oz. trout fillets
- 1 fresh lemon
- pinch salt
- pepper, to taste
- 1 cup shelled pistachios, crushed.

Direction:

Preheat the oven to 350°F. Pat fillets with paper towels. Put the skin-side down on an oiled baking sheet. Squeeze the juice of the lemon onto the skinless side. Sprinkle with salt and pepper. Add the pistachios to a blender or food processor and pulse five to seven times until they make a coarse, breadcrumb-like texture.

Garlicky Kale and Pea Sauté

It contains 3g of fat, 11g of carbohydrates, 5g of protein, and 85 calories.

Time: 10 minutes

Servings: 2 servings

Ingredients:

- 2 sliced garlic cloves
- 1 chopped hot red chili.
- 2 tablespoons of olive oil.
- 2 bunches of chopped kale.
- 1 lb. frozen peas.

Direction:

Mix all the ingredients except the peas in a saucepot. Cook the kale until it becomes tender for about 6 minutes. Add the peas and cook for an extra 2 minutes.

Blueberry, Peach, and Avocado Salad

It contains 8g of fat, 16g of carbohydrates, 2g of protein, and 130 calories.

Time: 45 minutes

Servings: 6 servings

Ingredients:

- 1 tablespoon of extra virgin olive oil
- 1 tablespoon of lime juice
- ½ teaspoon of lime zest
- ¼ teaspoon of salt
- 2 cups of fresh blueberries
- 1 avocado, pitted and cubed
- 2 large ripe peaches, pitted and cubed
- 1 tablespoon of finely chopped fresh basil.

Direction:

Whisk olive oil, lime juice, lime zest, and salt until well blended in a large bowl. Add blueberries, peaches, basil, and avocado. Combine properly and serve.

IVAN BURROWS

DINNER RECIPES

Salmon and Tomatoes

It contains 12g of fat, 3g of carbohydrates, 21g of protein, and 200 calories.

Time: 25 minutes

Servings: 4 servings

Ingredients:

- 2 tablespoons of avocado oil
- 4 boneless salmon fillets
- 1 cup of halved cherry tomatoes
- 2 chopped spring onions
- ½ cup of vegetable stock
- salt and black pepper
- ½ teaspoon of dried rosemary

Direction:

Combine fish with oil and other ingredients in a roasting pan. Put in the oven at 400°F and bake for 25 minutes. Divide between plates and serve.

Cauliflower Steak with Sweet-Pea Puree

It contains 4g of fat, 40g of carbohydrates, 15g of protein, and 235 calories.

Time: 35 minutes

Servings: 2 servings

Ingredients:

- 2 heads of cauliflower
- 1 teaspoon of olive oil
- ¼ teaspoon of paprika1 teaspoon of coriander
- ¼ teaspoon of black pepper sweet-pea puree
- 10 ounces of frozen green peas
- 1 onion, chopped
- 2 tablespoons of fresh parsley
- ¼ cup of unsweetened soy milk

Direction:

Preheat the oven to 425°F. Remove the bottom core of the cauliflower. Stand it on its base, beginning in the middle, and slice it in half. Then, slice the steaks about ¾ inches thick. Utilize a baking pan and set it in the steaks. Coat the front and back of the steak with olive oil. Sprinkle with coriander, paprika, and pepper. Bake for 30 minutes, flipping once.

Steam the chopped onions and peas until they are soft.

Put the vegetables in a blender with milk and parsley, and blend until smooth.

Black Bean Stuffed Sweet Potato

It contains 16g of fat, 53g of carbohydrates, 11g of protein, and 387 calories.

Time: 80 minutes

Servings: 4 servings

Ingredients:

- 4 sweet potatoes
- 15 ounces of cooked black beans
- ¼ teaspoon of ground black pepper
- ½ red onion, peeled and diced
- ½ teaspoon of sea salt
- ¼ teaspoon of onion powder
- ¼ teaspoon of garlic powder
- ¼ teaspoon of red chili powder
- ¼ teaspoon of cumin
- 1 teaspoon of lime juice
- 1-1/2 tablespoon of olive oil
- ½ cup of cashew cream sauce

Direction:

Spread the potatoes on a baking tray greased with oil, and bake for 65 minutes at 350°F until tender. In the meantime, prepare the sauce by whisking together the cream sauce, black pepper, and lime juice until combined. Then set it aside for now.

When is remaining 10 minutes are left for the baking time of the potatoes, heat the skillet pan with oil. Add in onion to cook until it's golden for 5 minutes.

Stir in spice, and cook for an extra 3 minutes. Stir in beans until combined, and cook for 5 minutes until hot.

Let the roasted sweet potatoes cool for 10 minutes, then cut them open, mash the flesh, and top with bean mixture, cilantro, and avocado. Then, drizzle with cream sauce, and serve right away.

Turkey-Ginger Sliders

This recipe can be used to make healthier burgers, meatballs, and appetizers.

It contains 14g of fat, 33g of carbohydrates, 25g of protein, and 350 calories.

Time: 30 minutes

Servings: 6 sliders

Ingredients:

- 10 ounces of 95% lean ground turkey
- 1 (1 inch) piece of ginger, sliced
- 1 shallot, minced
- 1 tablespoon of tomato paste
- salt and pepper, to taste
- 1 medium-sized cucumber, sliced on the diagonal
- 2 teaspoons of extra virgin olive oil
- 6 whole-grain slider buns

Direction:

Combine the turkey, ginger, shallot, and tomato paste in a medium-sized bowl. Season with salt and pepper. Mix until well combined. Form six patties, about ¼ inch thick.

Heat the olive oil in a medium pan on medium-high heat until it is hot. Add patties and cook for 1 to 2 minutes per side or until cooked through. Transfer to a paper towel-lined plate to drain. Assemble sliders by placing cucumber slices and patties between buns.

Roasted Halibut with Spicy Black Bean Cake

It contains 17g of total fat, 38g of carbohydrates, 31g of protein, and 430 calories.

Time: 1 hour 50 minutes

Servings: 8 servings

Ingredients:

Bean cakes

- 4 tablespoons of extra virgin oil, divided
- 1 white onion, peeled and diced
- 2 tablespoons of garlic cloves, crushed and chopped
- ¼ cup of jalapeño peppers stemmed and minced
- 2 teaspoons of toasted ground cumin
- 3 cups of cooked black beans, divided
- 1 teaspoon of kosher salt
- 1 teaspoon of ground pepper
- 2 cups of sweet potatoes, peeled and grated
- 2 eggs, lightly beaten

- ¾ cup of whole grain toasted breadcrumbs, plus extra for coating finished cakes

Halibut

- 2 pounds halibut fillet, skinned and portioned into 4-ounce pieces
- salt and pepper, to taste
- 1 tablespoon of toasted ground fennel seed
- ¼ cup of extra-virgin oil
- 1 lime, quartered to serve

Direction:

For the bean cakes, heat 2 tablespoons of olive oil in a small skillet over medium heat. Cook onion until it is soft, for about 1 minute. Then, stir in garlic, jalapeños, and toasted cumin. Cook for about 2 minutes until fragrant.

Transfer the contents of the skillet to a large bowl. Stir in 2 cups of cooked black beans and mash them with a fork. Season with salt and pepper. Add sweet potatoes, eggs, remaining 1 cup of cooked black beans, and breadcrumbs. Mix again to combine, and allow to chill for 30 minutes.

Divide into 16 small bowls and flatten into square patties. Use 2 tablespoons of olive oil to lightly grease the baking sheet. Dip patties into the breadcrumbs to coat and put on the oiled sheet pan, and allow to chill for 20 minutes. Preheat the oven to 450°F. Then, put the bean cakes in an oven and roast for 10 minutes or until the cake is slightly brown.

In the meantime, pat the halibut fillets dry with paper towels. Sprinkle salt, pepper, and fennel seeds to season the halibut portions. Heat ¼ cup of olive oil over medium heat in a large oven-proof pan until hot but not smoking. Put the halibut pieces into the pan and cook until the bottom side is golden and the edges of the fish start to look opaque, for about 3 minutes.

Toss the fish fillets over and put them in the oven for about 2 to 3 minutes or until the fillets are opaque in the center.

Serve the fish with warm roasted black bean cakes and fresh lime wedges.

Raspberry, Sriracha, and Ginger Glazed Salmon

The glazed salmon (which includes 1 ounce of glaze) contains 13g of fat, 14g of carbohydrates, 33g of protein, and 310 calories.

The Raspberry sriracha ginger glaze contains 0g of total fat, 14g of carbohydrates, 1g of protein, and 60 calories.

Time: 30 minutes

Servings: 8 servings

Ingredients:

Salmon

- 4 (5-ounce) salmon fillets
- 2 teaspoons extra-virgin olive oil
- 1 teaspoon of salt
- pepper to taste

Raspberry, Sriracha Ginger Glaze

- 4 ounces or 1 cup of ginger, peeled and sliced ¼ inch thick
- 4 cups of frozen raspberries, thawed

- 1 cup of mirin

- 1 cup of apple juice

- 1 cup of water

- 1-2 teaspoons (adjust heat to the desired level) of sriracha sauce

Direction:

Preheat the oven to 400°F. Then, season the salmon with olive oil, salt, and pepper, and set aside.

Prepare the raspberry sriracha ginger glaze. Combine all the ingredients in a medium saucepan and cook over medium heat. Bring to a boil, reduce the heat, and simmer until the liquid is reduced to at least 1/3 and slightly thickened. (Note: the sriracha sauce increases in heat level when the sauce is reduced.) Remove from heat and strain through a fine-mesh strainer into two small-sized bowls.

Brush the first set of the raspberry sriracha ginger glaze onto the seasoned salmon portions before baking. Put the salmon fillets on a baking sheet and place them in an oven. Let it bake for about 8 to 12 minutes until the salmon is done.

At the end of the baking, before serving, brush the second set of glaze on the salmon. Use ½ to 1 ounce of glaze per salmon portion.

Spaghetti with Chickpeas Meatballs

It contains 4g of fat, 63g of carbohydrates, 15g of protein, and 323 calories.

Time: 40 minutes

Servings: 8 servings

Ingredients:

- ½ cup of breadcrumbs
- 1 teaspoon of Italian seasoning
- 3 cups of chickpeas, drained and rinsed
- ½ teaspoon of salt
- 3 tablespoons of flaxseed, ground
- 2 teaspoons of onion powder
- 8 tablespoons of water
- ½ tablespoon of garlic powder
- ¼ cup of nutritional yeast
- 1 lb. of spaghetti
- 25 ounces of pasta sauce

Direction:

Preheat the oven to 325°F. Put the flax seeds in a bowl of water and set it aside for 5 minutes. Put the chickpeas and sat in a food processor and process them for 1 minute or until you get a smooth mixture. Then, transfer the chickpea mixture and flaxseed mixture into a large mixing bowl. Stir well. Once combined, add the remaining ingredients required to the bowl.

Stir everything until they are combined well enough. Then, make balls out of this mixture and arrange them on a parchment paper-lined baking sheet while leaving enough space in between. Bake for 33 to 35 minutes, Turn them once halfway through. Meanwhile, make the spaghetti according to the instructions on the packet. Cook until al dente. Put the spaghetti on the plate and top it with the meatballs and pasta sauce, then serve.

Walnut Salmon Mix

It contains 14g of fat, 3g of carbohydrates, 36g of protein, and 276 calories.

Time: 10 minutes

Servings: 4 servings

Ingredients:

- 4 salmon fillets, boneless
- 2 tablespoons of avocado oil
- Salt
- black pepper
- 1 tablespoon of lime juice
- 2 chopped shallots
- 2 tablespoons of chopped walnuts.
- 2 tablespoons of chopped parsley.

Direction:

Pour oil into the pan and heat over medium heat. Add shallots, stir, and sauté for 2 minutes. Add the fish and other ingredients and cook for 6 minutes on each side. Divide between plates and serve.

Chicken Thighs and Grapes Mix

It contains 12g of fat, 10g of carbohydrates, 34g of protein, and 289 calories.

Time: 42 minutes
Servings: 4 servings

Ingredients:

- 2 garlic cloves, chopped
- 1 cup of tomatoes, cubed
- 1 yellow onion, sliced
- black pepper
- ¼ cup of chicken stock, low-sodium
- 1 lb. chicken thighs
- 1 carrot, cubed
- 1 tablespoon of olive oil
- 1 cup of green grapes.

Direction:

Grease your baking pan with oil and arrange the chicken thighs inside. Add the other ingredients on top. Bake at 390°F for 40 minutes. Then, divide between plates and serve.

Moussaka

It contains 27g of fat, 46g of carbohydrates, 41g of protein, and 577 calories.

Time: 20 minutes

Servings: 2 servings

Ingredients:

- 1 tablespoon olive oil
- ½ onion, finely chopped
- 1 garlic clove, finely chopped
- 9 oz. lean beef mince
- 1 cup chopped tomatoes
- 1 tablespoon tomato purée
- 1 teaspoon ground cinnamon
- 1 cup can of chickpeas
- ⅔ cup feta cheese, crumbled
- dried mint
- brown bread, to serve

Direction:

Heat your oil in a pan and add onions and garlic. Fry until they turn soft. Add the mince and fry for 3-4 minutes until they turn brown. Tip the tomatoes into the pan and stir in the tomato purée and cinnamon. Then, season. Allow the mince to simmer for 20 minutes. Then, add chickpeas halfway through. Sprinkle the mint and feta over the mince. Serve with toasted bread.

Salmon with Potatoes and Corn Salad

It contains 21g of fat, 27g of carbohydrates, 43g of protein, and 479 calories.

Time: 30 minutes

Servings: 2 servings

Ingredients:

- 1 ⅓ cups baby new potatoes
- 1 sweetcorn cob
- 2 skinless salmon fillets
- ⅓ cup tomatoes

For the dressing:

- 1 tablespoon of red wine vinegar.
- 1 tablespoon extra-virgin olive oil.
- bunch of spring onions/scallions, finely chopped.
- 1 tablespoon capers, finely chopped.
- handful of basil leaves.

Direction:

Boil the potatoes until tender, and add corn for the final 5 minutes. Drain and allow to cool.

For the dressing, mix vinegar, oil, spring onions/scallions, basil, capers, and season.

Heat grill to high.

Rub some of the dressing on the salmon and cook it skinned-side down for 7 to 8 minutes. Add the salmon and drizzle over the remaining dressing.

Almond-Crusted Baked Salmon

It contains 17g of fat, 4g of carbohydrates, 29g of protein, and 290 calories.

Time: 20 minutes

Servings: 4 servings

Ingredients:

- 2 tablespoons Dijon mustard
- zest of 1 lemon
- 1 tablespoon chopped herbs of choice (dill, lemon thyme, chives, parsley)
- 4/6 oz. thick-cut salmon fillets
- Pepper
- ¼ cup of chopped almonds.

Direction:

Preheat the oven to 400°F. Mix the mustard, zest, and herbs on a plate. Pepper the salmon, dip in the mustard zest-herb mixture, then roll in the crushed almond and put in the oven for 10 minutes. Cover and let rest for 5 minutes. If you do not want to stain your blender, you can put nuts in a plastic sandwich bag and crush them with a rolling pin or the bottom of a cup. Rub the almonds onto the exposed side of the fish and transfer the pan to the oven. Bake for 20 to 25 minutes or until fish flakes easily with a fork. You can also transfer the fish to the broiler for the last couple of minutes of cooking to brown almonds.

Spicy Tomato Baked Egg

It contains 17g of fat, 45g of carbohydrates, 19g of protein, and 417 calories.

Time: 20 minutes

Servings: 2 servings

Ingredients:

- 1 tablespoon of olive oil
- 2 red onions, chopped
- 1 red chili, deseeded & chopped
- 1 garlic clove, sliced
- small bunch of coriander, stalks, and leaves chopped separately
- 4 cups cherry tomatoes
- 4 eggs
- brown bread, to serve

Direction:

Pour oil into a frying pan and cover with a lid. Then, cook the onions, garlic, chili, and coriander stalks for 5 minutes until they become soft.

Stir in the tomatoes and simmer for 8 to 10 minutes. Make 4 dips in the sauce with the back of a large spoon, then crack an egg into each one. Cover the pan with a lid and let it cook over low heat for 6 to 8 minutes until the egg is cooked to your liking. Then, scatter with the coriander leaves and serve with bread.

Five-Spice Chicken Breast

It contains 9g of fat, 5g of carbohydrates, 31g of protein, and 244 calories.

Time: 30 minutes

Servings: 4 servings

Ingredients:

- black pepper
- 1 teaspoon of five-spice
- 1 tablespoon of hot pepper
- 1 tablespoon of avocado oil
- 1 tablespoon of cilantro, chopped
- 2 chicken breast halves, skinless, deboned and halved
- 1 cup of tomatoes, crushed
- 2 tablespoons of coconut aminos.

Direction:

Pour oil into the pan and heat with medium heat. Then, add the meat and brown it for 2 minutes on each side. Add the tomatoes, five-spice, and other ingredients, and bring to a simmer to cook with medium heat for 30 minutes. Divide the whole mix between plates and serve.

SNACKS, SIDES, AND SPREADS

Basic Salsa

Salsa contains naturally wholesome fruits and vegetables, which add fresh and zesty flavors without an overload of sugar, salt, and saturated fat. Salsa is easy to make, and it goes with everything. It incorporates one of the MIND healthy foods for the brain, which is vegetables.

It contains 0g of fat, 8g of carbohydrates, 1g of protein, and 30 calories.

Time: 10 minutes to prepare and 1 hour to chill (optional)
Servings: 4 servings (1/4 cup each)

Ingredients:

- 3 Roma tomatoes, diced
- 1 medium sweet onion, diced
- ¼ cup of chopped, fresh cilantro, rinsed, and pat dry with paper towels
- 3 limes, juiced
- salt and pepper, to taste

Direction:

Combine the tomatoes, onion, cilantro, and lime juice. Add salt and pepper to taste. Also, keep in mind that the flavor will develop over time.

Collard Greens with Mustard Seeds

This recipe combines collard greens with flavorful apple cider vinegar, mustard seeds, and olive oil. Collards contain calcium-rich cruciferous vegetables that are packed with vitamins A and C.

It contains 7g of fat, 3g of carbohydrates, 1g of protein, and 75 calories.

Time: 23 minutes

Servings: 4 servings

Ingredients:

- 2 tablespoons of extra-virgin oil
- 1 small yellow onion, sliced
- 1 clove of garlic, minced
- 1 tablespoon of mustard seeds
- 1 bunch of collard greens sliced into ribbons
- 2 tablespoons of apple cider vinegar
- 2 tablespoons of water

Direction:

Add olive oil and onions to a medium sauté pan, and sauté for about 5 minutes. Then, add garlic and sauté until it is light brown. Add mustard seeds to the onion and garlic mixture, and shake them in the pan until they pop, about a minute or so. Put the collard greens into the sauté pan and add apple cider vinegar and water. Cover for 7 to 10 minutes. Then, serve immediately.

Oat Cranberry Pilaf with Pistachios

It contains 5g of total fat, 26g of carbohydrates, 8g of protein, and 170 calories.

Time: 40 minutes

Servings: 8 servings

Ingredients:

- 1 teaspoon of extra-virgin olive oil
- 1 small yellow onion, diced
- 3 stalks of celery with leaves, diced
- 1 clove of garlic, minced
- ½ cup of chopped mushrooms
- 2 tablespoons of chopped, fresh parsley
- ¼ teaspoon of ground turmeric
- 1 teaspoon of ground marjoram
- ½ teaspoon of pepper
- ½ cup of pistachios shelled
- 1 cup of canned whole cranberries
- 2 cups of vegetable broth
- 1-1/2 cups of old-fashioned oats

Direction:

Heat the oil in a large cast iron skillet. Add onion, celery, and garlic and sauté for 5 minutes. Add mushrooms, parsley, turmeric, marjoram, pepper, and pistachios, and sauté for extra 3 minutes.

Heat the oven to 350°F while the vegetable is cooking. Add cranberries, oats, broth, and oats to the skillet. Stir until smooth. Transfer skillet to oven and bake on top of the rack for 25 minutes, until it is golden and tender.

Lentils Spread

It contains 8g of fat, 60g of carbohydrates, 26g of protein, and 416 calories.

Time: 15 minutes

Servings: 4 servings

Ingredients:

- 2 cloves of garlic, minced
- ½ cup of cilantro, chopped
- 14 ounces of canned lentils, drained, unsalted, and rinsed
- 1 lemon juice
- 2 tablespoons of olive oil

Direction:

Combine the lentils, oil, and other ingredients in a blender. Pulse well, divide into bowls, and serve as a spread.

Roasted Walnuts

It contains 30g of fat, 6g of carbohydrates, 12g of protein, and 311 calories.

Time: 15 minutes

Servings: 8 servings

Ingredients:

- 14 ounces of walnuts
- ½ teaspoon of garlic powder
- 1 tablespoon of avocado oil
- ½ teaspoon of chili powder
- ½ teaspoon of smoked paprika
- ¼ teaspoon of cayenne pepper

Direction:

Spread the walnuts on the lined baking sheet. Add paprika and the other ingredients. Flip and bake at 410°F for 15 minutes. Divide into bowls and serve as a snack.

BEVERAGES AND
DESSERTS

Oat Milk

Oat milk is a mild-tasting dairy alternative that is simple and affordable to prepare at home. It contains MIND healthy foods for the brain, like whole grains.

It contains 5g of fat, 5g of carbohydrates, 1g of protein, and 30 calories.

Time: 5 to 10 minutes, 1hr chilling time

Servings: 4 servings

Ingredients:

- 4 cups of water
- 1 cup of quick-cooking oats (aka rolled, regular, instant, old fashioned.)
- 2 Medjool dates, pitted
- 1 teaspoon of vanilla extract
- pinch of salt

Direction:

Bring water to a simmer in a small pot, then add all ingredients to cook for 5 minutes. Then, blend all the ingredients in a blender or food processor until combined.

Strain through a fine mesh sieve over a large bowl, reserving the oats solids to use in soups, smoothies, or oatmeal.

Repeat the straining process if desired. Store in a jar with a lid. Chill for at least an hour and shake before serving.

Blueberry Banana Ice Cream

This recipe does not need added sugar, and it is good for brain health.

It contains 1g of total fat, 35g of carbohydrates, 2g of protein, and 140 calories.

Time: 5 minutes, 2 hours advanced freezing time for bananas

Servings: 4 servings

Ingredients:

- 2 frozen bananas, chopped
- 1 cup of frozen blueberries
- 2 vanilla beans, split lengthwise

Direction:

Chop and peel the bananas before freezing them. Freeze for at least 2 hours ahead of time. Add the bananas and blueberry inside a blender or food processor. Scrap vanilla seeds in from the beans and process or blend until creamy. Scoop into bowls and serve.

References

The MIND diet: A Scientific Approach to Enhancing Brain Function and Helping Prevent Alzheimer's and Dementia by Maggie Moon.

The MIND diet cookbook and Meal Plan by Eva Evans.

Lyssie Lakatos and Tammy Lakatos Shames from www.nutritiontwins.com

Sharon Palmer from www.sharonpalmer.com

Jessica Fishman from www.nutritioulicious.com.

The Bean Institute at www.beaninstitute.com

National Processed Raspberry Council from www.redrazz.org

Tracee Yablon Brenner from www.triadtowellness.com
US Highbush Blueberry Council from www.littlebluedynamos.com

Made in the USA
Monee, IL
29 September 2023